LIFE IS A GAME OF CONSEQUENCES

how and why we become ill

Dr Mollie Hunton

HOMOL PRESS

First published in 2020 by Homol Press.

Printed and bound by 4edge Limited, 22 Eldon Way Industrial Estate, Hockley, Essex, SS5 4AD.

ISBN: 978-1-5272-5135-9

Buy books and contact the author via homol@btinternet.com

Find this book under the section: Health, Medical

To all my family and friends

FOREWORD

This is a book about joined-up medicine, and how and why we become ill. I want to make a case for holism in medicine. At present, the system is one of rationalism. Rationalism is the principle or habit of accepting that reason is the supreme authority in matters of opinion, belief, or conduct. Holism is the idea that systems and their properties should be viewed as wholes and not just a collection of parts. An example of rationalism is the fact that there are so many medical specialities, all looking at smaller and smaller individual parts of the body. No one doctor can seem to put it all together.

A patient consulted me about her granddaughter and told me that she had asthma, eczema and, now at the age of ten, had developed ulcerative colitis. She saw a paediatric respiratory physician for her asthma, a paediatric dermatologist for her eczema, and a paediatric gastroenterologist for her ulcerative colitis. None of them corresponded with one another, only with the GP. She saw a different GP every time. No one saw her as a whole. The treatment for her was to have steroids from time to time, specially for the asthma attacks and eczema, and for exacerbations of her ulcerative colitis. It was possible that she would have to stay on steroids in varying doses for the rest of her life, with all their attendant problems. No one seemed to think that this was going to cause side effects. No one took a long-term view of her health. One of the problems with conventional medicine seems to be that the short-term view is the best, as in the long-term it might be a different doctor that has to deal with the problem in the future. None of the doctors that this child had seen had ever found a common theme to her problems, particularly allergies to food. This is what dismays me.

It also seems that GPs can only deal with one symptom at a time. Why should patients only have one symptom to express their problem? Why should they be expected to be ill in standard ways, when everyone is different?

This book will tell you how and why we become ill. It will become obvious, and you might wonder why no one has thought of the body in the way I explain before, but as long as we have a system of medicine that divides people into smaller and smaller groups, and labels them accordingly with diagnostic names, we will only know this name and not what the cause of the illness is. We then end up knowing what happens, that is, the symptoms, but not what caused them. It is only in recent years that we have had the knowledge to put everything together. As long as clinicians and researchers look at smaller and smaller parts of the body the question of cause will never be answered. Doctors should ask the patient what has made them ill and pay attention to the answer. If the doctor has difficulty with this situation it is because they have never learnt to see the patient as a whole. Every part of the human body is interconnected, and even one flaw in a certain part could set off a whole chain reaction to cause an illness.

The philosophy of rationalism says that reason alone is a source of knowledge and is independent of experience, whereas the theory of holism says that parts of a whole are an intimate interconnection, such that they cannot exist independently of the whole, or cannot be understood without reference to the whole, which is thus regarded as greater than the sum of parts. This is an anathema to conventional medicine.

Rationalism says that treating reason as the ultimate authority is the correct practice, but holism says that treating the whole person – taking into account their mental and social factors, rather than just the symptoms of disease – is the way forward.

Thomas Huxley said on reading Darwin: 'The best ideas are often staggeringly simple. How extremely stupid not to have thought of that!'

Each and every idea in this book has been researched, been – and continues to be – the subject of countless books and articles, and all areas of interest have their own experts. So there are lots of ideas about small and smaller things in the body but no one discipline to put them together. The idea is that if these individual processes can be understood a drug will be found to stop it when it goes wrong. Instead, the question should be: why has this happened in this patient at this time and how can it be healed, not suppressed.

Curiosity is the enemy of certainty. Doctors should be much more curious about their patients but have not the time or interest as it does not help with diagnosis, the only end point.

I hope to show in this book that doctors are missing the opportunity to truly heal people, rather than just suppressing the symptoms with medication, if they don't look at the whole person. This includes as we will see, their mental and emotional side. It would give doctors a huge insight into what makes the patient ill. Unfortunately, knowing about emotional and mental aspects of disease causes a real problem, as they have no way of tackling the situation. There is no medication available for this sort of thing. The only way they might help is to suggest psychological treatment, which usually involves a great deal of counselling, and time-consuming cognitive behavioural therapy (CBT), if it is available. There is a vast increase in the number of people with mental health problems and virtually no way to detect, treat, and monitor their progress. This reflects poorly on doctors' ability to cope with the problem, and this must be a result of *their* teachers' difficulties in understanding and passing on *their* knowledge. The inability to cope is a major part of becoming ill, so it is possible that many doctors will give up practising in the UK and go abroad, where they think that life will be easier.

Out of all the specialities there are in medicine, there are quite a few that do not involve much live-patient contact, like pathology, microbiology, biochemistry, anaesthetics, genetics, blood transfusions, forensic medicine, intensive care, and public health. If seeing patients is too difficult and anxiety-provoking for the doctor, he, or she, thinks about taking up another career outside medicine – or inside, but avoiding patient contact. This reflects a doctor as a technician. The most difficult thing about being a doctor is talking to people and trying to find out what is really wrong. To me that is the most interesting part of the job. I knew as soon as I had done my introductory course in homeopathy that this was the way forward for me. It put me on a different level in the consulting room, and stopped me just being a technician. I regret that modern medicine has reduced the body to small individual parts, and the concept that problems can be solved by attention to these parts only. I also regret that the attitude is for short-term gains with long-term problems, and for lack of continuity of care. There are no family doctors now. Seeing a different doctor each consultation is bound to cause consequences.

I have attempted to put the whole body together and therefore come across new ways of looking at life, like the inability to cope syndrome and the role of anxiety in all illness. I have also included patient histories, especially homeopathic, as this method always seems the most rational way of treating most disease.

I went to a wedding where the bride and groom had many friends who were junior doctors. At one point they were discussing what they were going to specialise in. Only one wanted to be a GP. The rest were talking about how they could make the most money from private practice and avoid a lot of night duty. It seems that being a doctor is no longer a vocation. However, the doctors and vets that I meet at homeopathic meetings still seem to have a desire to cure patients. I used to ask the medical students I taught to define 'cure', and we debated things such as: 'Would removing a cancer result in a cure?' Dr Samuel Friedrich Hahnemann, the founder of homeopathy, said that if you don't remove the cause, you never can cure a disease.

As doctors, we go into specialities that suit our personality – maybe subconsciously. That is why homeopathy suits me, as I feel the need to get to the root cause of why a patient becomes ill at a certain time in their lives. It also reflects our training. I feel sorry for young doctors now, as they have been through medical school without some of the benefits that we had. I feel that modern methods of teaching lack the human touch. You cannot learn anatomy from computer images; they are just a guide.

Through reading this book, I hope that you get more insight into your illness or condition if you're a patient, or insight into your patient and their illness or condition, if you're a doctor.

1

THE MEANING OF LIFE:
Population and Longevity

For the individual the meaning of life is to live happily and with satisfaction – a good life. Biologically, the meaning of our lives is to live and reproduce. If we reproduce too much the planet becomes overcrowded and people suffer either individually due to lack of jobs leading to poverty, housing and over population, or as nations with descent into war. If we do not reproduce successfully the population fails and the race dies out.

Several factors encourage disease such as overcrowding, lack of education and mental health problems. Consequently, the survival of the fittest applies to humans as well as to wild animals. In the 1960s an experiment was carried out with a male and female rat in a large cage. As the rats kept on reproducing and numbers grew, the problems grew correspondingly. Dominant males became aggressive, some moving in groups, attacking females and the young. Mating behaviours were disrupted with some becoming exclusively homosexual. Others became pansexual and hypersexual, attempting to mount any rat they encountered. Mothers neglected their infants, first failing to construct proper nests, and then abandoning or attacking their infants. In certain sections of the pens, infant mortality rose as high as 96%, with the dead being cannibalised by adults. Subordinate animals withdrew psychologically, surviving in a physical sense but at an immense psychological cost. These rats were the majority in the late phases of growth, existing as a vacant, huddled mass in the centre of the cage. Unable to breed, the population plummeted and did not recover. The crowded rodents had lost their ability to coexist harmoniously, even after the population numbers once again fell to a low level. At a certain density, they had ceased to act like rats, the changes being permanent. As the population grew, this became increasingly problematic. As the cages heaved with animals, one of the scientists conducting the experiment described rodent 'utopia' as having become 'hell'. It was inevitable that the colony of rats would be compared to human overcrowding.

People are all different as a result of their genes, their upbringing, the development of their brains and how it is wired up, which in turn depends on nutrition. The old 'nature versus nurture' idea made us think about the relationship between genetic programming and the functioning of the brain with patterns that emerge due to conditioning. The development of computing has given us a view of the brain as a wired-up organ, functioning on electromagnetism (a branch of physics) as well as biochemistry.

Personality is the essence of the individual because it defines your behaviour in life and its consequences. Would people change their behaviour patterns if they realised the consequences? If you knew that you were similar to your paternal grandfather who had died from a heart attack, aged 61, after becoming very angry, would you consider changing your anger patterns? Is it more damaging if you keep your anger inside or let it out, which may in turn lead to a violent outcome?

Everyone has some anger inside them, and we can all be put on a linear scale somewhere for every emotion and every personality characteristic. Examples:

• Calmness, to anger

• Shy, to extrovert

• Reserved (lack of confidence), to confident

Good health is the most important thing in life as disablement may lead to an unfulfilled life. Since

Victorian times public health has educated us to live in a healthy way by providing us with clean water, sewerage and better housing. During the last century girls in particular have greatly benefited from much improved education. Modern statistics have produced information about the incidence of disease and its contributing factors. We all know, for example, that smoking can cause lung cancer, but not in everyone who smokes, because internal factors must also be involved. It is a reflection of the immune system not coping. Smoking is also a factor in other cancers, chronic obstructive pulmonary disease, peripheral vascular disease, and the complications of diabetes; and most other illnesses are worsened by smoking.

To look at the causes of disease we need to go back further in your personal time to see what altered your immune system.

Statistics take no account of a patient's individuality. This is also true of drug research which is only done on healthy, young males, and takes no account of gender or age, particularly children, the elderly, and women. They also take no account of weight. This is one of the reasons that so many people have side effects.

We have learnt to measure intelligence, and produced a bell-shaped normal distribution curve for populations in this country. The mean IQ is 100 in the UK. In some other countries it is just a little more or a little less. Most of our population is between 80 and 120 with those below 40 having severe learning difficulties, and those above 160 classed as geniuses. However, intelligence does not automatically produce insight as this is dependent on how that intelligence is used and developed from one's background. It is possible to have the attributes to run a successful business, but if you are manipulative or a bully your staff will be unhappy. If you don't realise or don't care, you will have frequent turnover of staff. Personality and intelligence need to work together.

Fewer children are born to educated women, which is a crucial factor in avoiding overpopulation. The question is whether a person's IQ is genetic and laid down at birth, or if it can it be improved. If the suggestion is that it cannot be altered then subsequent education is dependent upon what is present at birth and cannot be developed further. However, personality is your essence – whether you're hard-working, inventive and thoughtful, or lazy and shy, for example – and is developed during early life by the events around you. Rudolph Steiner used this model in his schools to develop pupils' natural talents.

Population

There has been a preponderance of children in the world until recently, but in 2017 the average age of people became 30, a figure which is on an upward trend. In 2050 it is estimated that it will be 38. This will mean there will be fewer children in the world and an ageing population. However, this trend may not necessarily continue.

If there are large numbers of young people, as happened with the baby boom following World War II, there are both problems and opportunities within society. If young people are unable to get jobs there will be unrest appearing in various ways. Large numbers of dependent elderly people cause crises in healthcare, but once the present generation of elders is gone, there will be fewer and fewer to replace them, because the many unhealthy people of today may not live as long.

The more you educate women the fewer children they have. At present the birth rate is 1.5 children per woman in China, and 1.8 in the UK and falling. If the population is not replaced it will decline. Young people in the UK are struggling, with a huge increase in incidences of cancer, chronic disease, and mental health problems. They are in debt if they go away to university so tend to live with their parents, which can be stressful for everyone. We are not alone in the UK. In Japan young people also go home to live with their parents after university because housing is so expensive. They are tending to not marry or have relationships, and so are not having children. The birth rate has dropped to a very low level, so the indicators are towards a declining population with fewer children who are less healthy. The decrease of marriages has obviously had an impact on the rate of reproduction, which becomes a vicious circle.

Infant Mortality Rate

2,900 infants under the age of one die in Britain annually. On the worldwide scale, Singapore has the lowest infant mortality rate, with Sweden second, and Japan third. The UK is 25th, and the worst is the USA at 34th.

There is a positive correlation between vaccine schedules, the number of vaccines given, and infant mortality, including sudden infant death syndrome. The least vaccinated children are from Sweden, Iceland and Japan, with 12 given in the first year of life. Singapore gives 17, the UK 19, and the USA 26.

Doctors

If the population does decline, there will not be the need to have quite so many doctors. There used to be under 100 medical students in each year. Now there are 400. It is possible to go through medical school now and not meet all your classmates. To avoid building bigger medical schools, students are sent out to general practice, which in turn means that GPs who teach students have less time to see their patients. This also happens with GPs who become managers in their own practices or work on local Clinical Commissioning Group committees, which also means less time to see their patients. Practices then have to take on more doctors to cope with the same number of patients.

Young doctors have less experience in general medicine as they see fewer patients in hospitals due to working shorter shifts in hospital than previously. They do not see the range of patients as junior doctors used to. Consequently, entering general-practice doctors are inexperienced and ill-prepared, which can be daunting for some, and the process of sorting patients' problems out takes longer. The undergraduates often seem to lack confidence and the maturity to deal with the serious situations that arise in medicine. Consequently, they feel anxious and lose confidence. There is a high incidence of mental health problems in medical students. Despite the changes in working shifts and not being 'on call', they appear to be stressed and tired. A lot of them feel stressed enough to consider that practising in another country would be easier and would like to emigrate.

Fertility

By 2050 the most populous countries will be China, Nigeria and the USA. There will be birth surges in Kenya, Uganda and Ethiopia.

At present fertility rates are declining all over the world. Japan's population is expected to fall by 30% over the next 40 years. Only 2% of their children are born to single mothers. Japanese women are now more educated and therefore less compliant, which men see as a threat to their relationships. Apparently, this is causing a rise of 'virtual love', which many prefer to complex relationships and actual physical fulfilment.

According to the UK's Office for National Statistics, in 2014 more than 35% of people were not married or had never been married. This is the lowest since records began and is a contributing factor in the housing crisis. Those people who are single either from choice, divorced or widowed all wish to live in their own property.

Despite the prophecy that many people will live to be 100 as appears to be happening at the present time, and possibly even 120, this figure may not be sustainable. Fewer people may live to be 100 as there is so much ill health amongst younger people today. The falling birth rate in the UK from 1.9 in 2010 to 1.88 in 2016 suggests the rising average age of people will be due to fewer children.

Young people in the UK are struggling. They have an increased incidence of severe mental health problems, cancers and chronic diseases. There are more babies born with abnormalities, stillbirths and severe prematurity than ever before. All the indicators point to a decline in health, and by the time the current cohort of young people become of pensionable age, there will be considerably fewer of them than there are today.

We have a vicious circle of fewer children who are less healthy, fewer marriages, more fertility problems, more people with severe illnesses and disabilities, and more with chronic illnesses, thus a decline in population.

The graph below shows this. After a steep increase in the population, during the Industrial Revolution, it reaches a peak, where we are now, and then levels off. A decline follows, which would reduce the UK population to pre-Revolution numbers. This only applies to the indigenous population and not to recent immigrants, probably people who are escaping the effects of global warming, as they may not be affected by the same things that affect us.

The left side of the graph is a solid line because it reflects measured levels of population. The right-hand side is a dotted line because it is a projected outcome using information available at present and following the mathematical model of a bell-shaped curve.

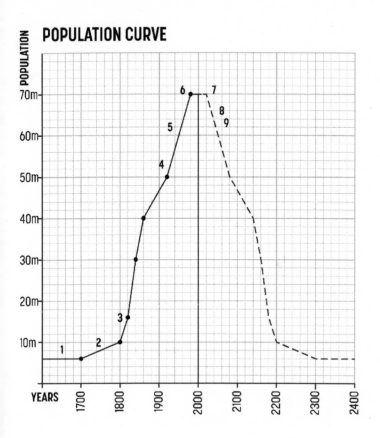

POPULATION CURVE

Key:

1. Before 1700: Apart from wars, the biggest killers of adults were epidemics of cholera, diphtheria, plague and typhus, and common infections in children. Personal hygiene and household cleanliness were non-existent in poor families. The only people to turn to during illness were women who used herbal preparations. The population stayed steady at around six million in the UK.

2. After 1700: People started to move into towns and cities. It was not until Dr John Snow discovered the origins of cholera in the water supplies, and Joseph Bazalgette built sewers, that public health became important and the population started to increase. Dr William Chamberlen and his sons took the subject of obstetrics seriously, and invented and used forceps that helped with obstructed labour. The maternal death rate started to fall, and with the introduction of hand-washing by Semmelweis to obstetrics, the maternal mortality also dropped. Many children still died in their first few years though, of things like scarlet fever and diphtheria.

3. Next came the Industrial Revolution, which gave people greater wealth. Consequently, malnutrition was less common so families grew larger and the population

increased rapidly. Life expectancy was around 42 years old in 1840 – the main killers being TB, the mining industry and smoking in men, childbirth complications and infections in women, and infectious diseases in children.

4. Then came two world wars with their horrendous death rates. Despite these and the subsequent influenza pandemic in 1919, the UK population still rose to 40 million. However, the rate of increase was slowing down, so much so that in the 1950s there were not enough people to take the available jobs. At this point immigrants from the West Indies were encouraged to come to the UK.

5. The twentieth century saw the growth of pharmaceutical business, with antibiotics being heralded as lifesavers. Modern drugs were evolving from herbal remedies, like willow bark used for pain, to laboratory manufactured compounds like acetyl salicylic acid, known as aspirin. When I was a junior doctor, I admitted a patient who needed digoxin to control his heart rate, but it made him vomit. The dose was reduced to the lowest amount available, but he was still sick. As the patient was reacting to the factory-made chemical, the consultant suggested he be given digitalis folia, the herbal variation

still available at that time. Not only did it help the cardiac rhythm, but his sickness stopped. Digitalis folia was, of course, eventually withdrawn, and if people now react badly to digoxin, they are given extra medication to counteract the vomiting.

6. Big pharma took a stranglehold on doctors and told them what to prescribe for everything. This happened from the discovery of penicillin onwards, when the latest wonder drug or update would be made available to GPs. We used to call this 'molecular roulette', and the reps would tell us that the latest version of an old drug was much better, as it was a more refined formula. The structure of the previous drug had been altered by a small amount of the molecule and the variation tested in mice. Clinical trials would then take place on healthy, young men who were not taking any medication. A lot of drugs, once released to the general public, caused so many side effects that they rapidly disappeared. Opren, medication for arthritis, is an example. The main problem with non-steroidal anti-inflammatories was, and still is, stomach bleeding. Opren capsules had a pinhole in the casing and when swallowed were supposed to pass through the stomach and release the medication lower down the bowel. Unfortunately, the bleeding then occurred in the

bowel, which was more serious, as it was difficult to localise. Opren was rapidly withdrawn.

It would appear that with modern medication you often get short-term relief and long-term problems. Why did so many haemophiliacs die of AIDS and hepatitis? Because of contaminated blood products. The NHS is paying out millions of pounds in compensation to people affected. It seems that the fittest people could be those who keep away from their doctors.

7. There are now fewer people reproducing themselves. Those who are gay or suffer with autism are unlikely to do so. More people than ever are dying at a young age. More people have a learning disability because of an increase in premature births. Women also may prefer careers to children and marriage.

8. Big business brings problems that have to be dealt with. Noxious chemicals are being put into our environment and the results are more diseases like asthma and strain on the immune system.

9. Society now has to contend with global warming, mining, deforestation and territory destruction by war and natural disasters like fires. The life to which we have

become accustomed will eventually run out of the resources we need to sustain it. Will there be enough food to feed everyone? The more people we try to feed, the more land becomes degraded and artificial chemicals have to be used.

The population is unhealthy, with increasing incidence of childhood cancer and serious chronic disease. People are damaged by alcohol, drugs, doctors, and medicines. There is famine in parts of the world and too much junk food in other countries. There are more people with severe learning difficulties, autism and mental health problems. The NHS cannot afford it all and cannot cope with the sheer number of ill people. People are too fond of their own ways of life to marry and have a family, or are unable to face the prospects of a job and mortgage, so the birth rate is declining.

We are definitely on the downward slope of the graph and unless it is understood what is happening, halt the destruction and mend the environment, the human race cannot survive.

The population growth curve was explained at a family-planning course I went to as a postgraduate. I found it a very vivid concept and have thought about it frequently since. My special interest in GP was in family planning because I strongly believed in the protection of women from the tyranny of childbirth and having large families. The lecturer pointed out that we were nearing the top of the rising curve, implying that there would be a period of levelling off before the population would decline sharply. I believe we are at the start of the decline which can be traced back to poor health initiated by big business and big pharma, and food manufacturers. Consumer industries such as cosmetics and cleaning materials are all putting noxious chemicals into the environment, which are damaging our health.

As a young doctor, I did a postgraduate job in paediatrics before there were sub-specialities. A paediatrician then looked after the health of all the children in the area. There were only two children with cancer, both of whom had leukaemia, and thus no need for children's cancer trusts and hospices. We now need paediatric oncologists and even they sub-specialise in the type of cancers they look after. Why have things changed? Today there are more of all diseases with more new diseases and neonatal defects to deal with. Hence there is now a need for so many specialities.

Why are people so ill and disabled and how can the people who work support all the people who do not?

Scotland is facing an unexpected and unprecedented mortality crisis according to newly released figures. They reveal that between 2013 and 2016 life expectancy failed to rise for the first time since records were published in 1861. More people died in 2015 than in any other single year since the Second World War. The rate was almost twice as high as in England and Wales. Between 2012 and 2015 the ages at which women and men in Scotland could expect to live remained static at 81.1 and 77.1 respectively. This is the first time in 150 years that life expectancy has not increased and suggests that the benefits to human longevity associated with better healthcare, education and housing as well as advances in medical technology and the fight against poverty are no longer effective in lengthening our lives. Life expectancy is going into reverse. It is also possible that we should expect a similar trend in the rest of the UK. This trend is not seen, at present, in other countries in Europe or elsewhere in the world.

There is mounting evidence of falls in life expectancy taking place within particular groups of society, associated with poverty, poor education, smoking and alcohol.

What we see in Scotland is despite the fact that public spending is higher per head than the UK average life expectancy is declining. I suggest that this trend will continue, as a consequence of our unsurmountable health problems.

Aldous Huxley said in the foreword to *Brave New World*:

It is only by means of the sciences of life that the quality of life can be changed. The sciences can be applied in such a way that they will destroy life or make the living of it impossibly complex.

We need to take heed of this prophecy.

2

MODERN MEDICINE CAN BE A HEALTH HAZARD:

Iatrogenic Disease

When I was a student, a question in the medicine paper in our finals asked: 'What do you understand by the term iatrogenic disease?' The invigilator had to tell us that iatrogenic meant 'caused by the doctor', as no one had come across the word. They were inviting us to write what we knew about drug side effects and other mishaps in medicine and surgery. Iatrogenic disease was very uncommon.

Now it is very common. All drug side effects are caused by the inability to foretell how the patient will react, but the patient trusts the doctor and consents to take the medication often without thinking that there may be consequences. However, we now also have to take into consideration errors of omission which means something has been missed and usually results from not listening and missing a diagnosis. Errors of commission occur when you entrust your body to a physician, surgeon or nurse and they do not perform the task as it should be done, which includes forgetting to refer patients, not reading results, information going missing, the wrong limb operated upon and so forth.

Iatrogenic Deaths

The list is alarmingly long, but the causes are the same in the USA and UK, and consist of chemotherapy, hospital errors, drug-resistant TB, bedsores, hospital malnutrition, adverse drug reactions like allergies, medical errors (missed diagnoses, surgery to the wrong part), hospital infections like MRSA and C. difficile, drug-resistant infections like pseudomonas, enterobacter, streptococci, salmonella, and shigella. Drugs like barbiturates and SSRIs (selective serotonin reuptake inhibitors) taken for depression, other antidepressants and tranquillisers, and opioids: morphine, codeine and heroin. Most other drugs, especially in combinations – not prescribing the correct medication, for example, or failing to estimate the severity of illness, and not prescribing steroids for asthma attacks. Legal abortions; retention of foreign objects, usually associated with surgery.

29

These are only the deaths. The children and adults with damaged health are not recorded.

Now hospitals have large departments, with many employees to deal with all the complaints. The system has to pay out a lot of money to people who have been damaged – the most recent being people with haemophilia, boys and men in the 1980s who were damaged by the system not providing healthy factor VIII replacement injections. These were needed to enable the blood to clot properly, but were made from pooled blood products, imported from the USA. It was not known at the time, but these products were full of viruses like hepatitis and HIV, which were passed on to the recipients, who then developed the diseases and usually died.

When I was a junior doctor, errors by doctors such as surgical mistakes were very rare. If one did occur, no matter whichever member of the team had caused it, be it junior or senior house officer, the registrar, the senior registrar, or the consultant, it was the consultant who saw the patient and discussed it. Consequently, very few people complained, and there was no need for a complaints department.

The problem nowadays is on a different level. Junior doctors seem to suffer a lot from lack of confidence, exhaustion, ignorance and an inability to see the consequences of their actions as well as some of them having language-barrier problems.

Doctors also now work shifts, whereas we worked one in two, i.e., 36 hours on, 12 hours off. As a junior doctor I had to live-in, so to be on call. The doctors' and nurses' residences were sold off or put to other uses when new contracts were developed. There was no official postgraduate training, but you learnt from listening to your superiors and, of course, from experience.

By the time I graduated I had already done locums for house officers in the year above me. When I started work, I looked after two wards, with 30 patients in each (or 35 plus on a busy admitting day). When on call I also looked after another two wards belonging to the other consultant physician. That was up to 120 patients plus admitting all the emergencies from local GPs. I saw patients with every category of disease from myocardial infarction to malignant hypertension, acute leukaemia and septicaemia. There were no coronary care or intensive care units and the physicians and surgeons were generalists. So I had a huge amount of experience by the time I registered.

However, specialisation has meant that new techniques have been developed for the care of people with life-threatening problems, much to the benefit of the patient.

When I was on call the GP would ring up to ask for the patient to be admitted and would send a letter with helpful information about the patient, which saved a lot of time. I was not allowed to refuse any patients and had to find a bed for them somewhere, even in the middle of the ward, which was laid out in the Nightingale style. That meant that the sister could keep an eye on the whole ward and if something was wrong could spot it at once. Now the nurses cluster round the computer on the nursing station which is often around a corner, out of sight. Consequently, the nurses can miss a lot of what goes on.

My consultant did ward rounds every day at 8.30 a.m. Afterwards, I ended up with a long list of tests that had to be done. There were no technicians to take blood or to do ECGs, etc., nor any ward staff to fill out forms.

Medical Education

The general consensus amongst retired doctors is that modern doctors are not as well grounded in basic sciences, e.g., anatomy, physiology, histology, pathology, haematology and microbiology as our generation was. This causes lack of confidence because of relative ignorance. This is what causes mistakes not tiredness. We made diagnoses confidently without scans and blood tests, took histories and examined patients as we had been taught. We had no paramedics to diagnose heart attacks before the patient got to the hospital.

The education of doctors and nurses has changed considerably in the last 50 years.

The Salmon Report took experienced nursing sisters off the wards into administration because that was the only way they could earn more money. Consequently, nurses who had been qualified for no more than a few years found themselves in charge of wards, with very little experience. Nursing was always a practical, hands-on vocation, but sending students to university and introducing technology and computers has changed things, especially the attitude to caring and hands on nursing. The more practical side of nursing is now done

33

by ward aides and cleaners. Nurses now consider themselves scientists. They specialise in single subjects as do the doctors and become specialist nurse practitioners. This is helpful to the doctor but may not always be to the patient if the nurse misses a diagnosis.

Medical students are now taught differently. Instead of learning the basics in the first 18 months, then doing exams in all those subjects before starting to see patients, they now see patients from the start of their training. As there are currently 400 students per year (politicians' efforts to increase the number of doctors), there are too many students for the medical school staff and buildings to cope with, so they are sent out to GP practices to see patients. Their learning becomes disease orientated, not patient orientated. The knock-on effect of this is that GPs teach undergraduates, and if you teach you are not seeing your own patients. As a consequence, GPs need to take on more partners, assistants, the recently qualified, part-timers, and GPs in training, to cope with the number of patients to be seen. It often means that patients rarely see the same doctor. Few follow-up appointments are made and trainee GPs move practices frequently. This all contributes to the problems within the NHS.

The number of locums employed has more than doubled since 2009 and there has been an annual rise of 12%, one reason being that GPs are no longer willing to do night duty.

Because of super specialisation and ward closures, young doctors do not see the range of illness that they used to. It must be hard to go into GP and not feel confident as a result of lack of experience. There are so many mental health problems suffered by young doctors who cannot cope that a special mental health service offering support has been set up.

Doctors now specialise in narrower and narrower fields. It must be difficult to work out on which ward your patients are staying as most wards take patients with all problems, and occasionally of mixed sex. One consultant used to look after the whole ward but now each patient has his own consultant in the speciality into which his illness fits. How do consultants know where their patients are? I have had patients over recent years who have been in hospital and not known which consultant looked after them as they did not see him (or her) all the time they were hospitalised. If the consultants are not on the wards seeing patients what are they doing? Outpatient clinics?

35

Meetings? Writing letters and reports? Seeing private patients? Our consultants looked after 70 patients on the wards, but now they may have no more than 10.

Hospitals face closure of wards as a result of having to find savings of £1 billion. A & E and maternity wards suffer most.

Diagnoses

Modern medicine is fairly good at diagnosis – that is, putting a name to a condition. For example, prion disease is due to proteinaceous infection particles which cause neurodegenerative disease like CJD (mad cow disease). Unfortunately, it is not good at curing. However, investigations can throw up more problems than they solve, as with mammograms, cervical smears and head and neck scans, which report changes that cannot be identified or diagnosed.

I was so concerned about the number of ladies with unidentified infections on their cervical smears that I asked the microbiologist if I could investigate them. She allowed me to swab 25 consecutive patients, of whom three had chlamydia, one had gonorrhoea, six had thrush, nine had non-specific virus infections, and six were undiagnosed. They were all treated, and had all cleared up at the one-year recall for the next smear, including the patients with minor virus changes. All were spared a visit to the gynaecologist as a year later their smears were normal. Now smears are taken by nurses and as long as there are no abnormal precancerous cells present, any infections are ignored. What a missed opportunity!

Mammograms and scans can show lesions that are uninterpretable, so need further investigations using procedures such as biopsies. Then decisions have to be made about treatment. Is there cancer present, one that is slow-growing, one that is likely to spread, or is there no cancer present at all? More problems may be caused than can be solved. Radiology reporting is now often outsourced to other countries as our consultants are so overloaded and computers are being programmed to interpret what is seen.

A patient with breast cancer which had been picked up on screening some years previously was having a lesion in her chest scanned to see if it was growing. Unfortunately, the one on her scapula which was growing more quickly was completely missed.

Modern medicine still looks at patients in categories, as a gut problem or joint problem. The human body is dynamic and should be looked at as a whole. Attempting to suppress symptoms with medication will only upset the body's balancing systems.

Medical Technology

The other 'problem' is inventions. Scans, for example, were invented in the 1960s and were used to try to detect how low-lying the placenta was in pregnant patients who had bleeds. Most of the other problems of childbirth were detectable by clinical examination. Now scans are relied on more than clinical skills, which lead to mistakes. An example of this was the non-examination of a lady after an emergency caesarean section, which had been performed for obstructed labour and foetal distress. As no one had assessed her pelvis, she was allowed to go into labour a second time, not knowing she had a narrow pelvis and could never deliver normally.

Despite the technology available patients with cancer are not diagnosed as early as they should be. Our local hospital was put in the 'needs improvement' category

(2016) with only 55% of patients receiving early diagnosis. The national standard is 87%. The aim is to achieve 75% one-year survival for all cancers by 2020, and for patients to be given a definite diagnosis or an all clear within 28 days of being referred by their GP. There is no mention of cure.

Problems also occur as a result of not seeing the same doctor each time, both at the GPs and at hospital. This problem is compounded by the use of computers. Many people complain to me that the doctor never looked at them, only the computer. On the computer doctors only have access to one page at a time, and therefore cannot see information from different sources at the same time. I used to be able to spread the patients' notes out across the desk so that results, letters, past history and current history could all be accessed easily. All notes were kept and not destroyed after a number of years in the same way that computer systems can delete records. The method of not following patients (who have had investigations) up is fraught with dire consequences as abnormal results can be easily missed. 'No news is good news' is a potentially unreliable method of working. If doctors work shifts and are not at work every day, the person who reads the results may not understand the significance of those results and what subsequent action may be needed.

Diagnoses depend on a number of factors: how early patients present, how skilful the doctor is at picking up the significance of the symptoms, making sure referrals do not get lost, and that communication with the patient is accurate and efficient.

Once admitted to hospital it is by no means clear that you will survive. Many factors are involved, such as poor communication between staff about nutrition, hospital superbugs, etc. Do staff pay attention to you when you have a problem? A patient went in to hospital for a prostatectomy for cancer. He suffered from atrial fibrillation and took warfarin. Before the surgery he was advised to stop the warfarin and was given heparin injections. His surgery went well, but when he came round, he realised he could not see properly. He told a nurse about it and she said that this was common after surgery and should improve. The next day it was still present and he told her again. This time he was told to be patient. No doctor visited him to speak about the problem. When he was ready for discharge, he had still not been able to discuss his symptoms with anyone. When he got home, he saw his GP and told him. Subsequently an outpatient appointment with another consultant took place and the patient was advised to have a brain scan. By the time he had the scan two months had passed and he still had half his vision in each eye missing. The scan showed a bleed in his optic chiasma as the cause of his loss of vision, and he is now disabled and cannot drive. He was perfectly fit before the surgery and now has difficulty getting around and has been registered as partially sighted. He exchanged the prospect of prostatic cancer for partial sight.

Hospital Infections

A young man aged 20 was a runner and fractured his ankle. He was admitted to the local hospital and had pin and plate surgery for the fracture. After a few days he ran a fever and complained of pain in the ankle with swelling and discharge through the wound. A swab showed MRSA and he was put on intravenous antibiotics.

Three weeks later I met his mum when out shopping. She told me about the situation and asked for help as she was frightened about his condition. He had had three weeks on

41

a drip, considerable loss of weight due to not eating, and was still running a temperature despite the antibiotics. He was faced with the threat of losing his foot if the infection could not be controlled. She was afraid he was going to die as he was so ill.

I gave her some homeopathic remedies – arnica 200C for injury, MRSA 200C for the infection, and symphytum 200C to heal the bones, and suggested he sucked one of each three times a day. I said she should discuss it with the consultant and I would be willing to go up and see him if he wanted me to. She went straight to the hospital and saw the consultant. He shrugged his shoulders and said that as he had no more ideas to suggest he didn't mind the homeopathic medication as he knew it would not interfere with any of the regular treatment.

On the following day he felt well enough to ask for food. His temperature had settled by the next day and on the third day the drip came down. He was discharged a few days later and made good progress. Some years later the plates caused further problems and they were removed. His foot was saved and he has been able to go back to running.

Cross Infection

Does hand-washing help, or clean clothes, or not wearing ward clothes outside the hospital? Should you keep your nails clean and neatly clipped with no varnish on them? (Things matrons used to be keen on.) Should doctors wear a bow tie rather than an ordinary one? When you lean forward does your long hair drop bacteria or viruses onto patients, or should you keep your hair off your face? When I did obstetrics and had long hair, the senior midwife made me plait it to keep it out of the way, and fringes were not allowed. Why has this sort of discipline disappeared? Why do doctors usually wear casual clothes and not white coats any more? There were rarely post-operative infections when the old rules applied.

Why do some doctors and nurses in theatres not cover their hair and noses? We had nasal swabs as students and were told which of us were carrying staphylococci. Those who were had to have some treatment. All surgeons, anaesthetists, and all theatre staff know about this problem, but you frequently see doctors operating (particularly on TV) with their noses uncovered and hair escaping from masks.

Keeping Up To Date

Up to 46,000 patients a year die because NHS treatments trail behind the best in the world. Why do our doctors not seem to know what goes on outside the UK? And why do we not learn from doctors in other countries, or share information with vets? I have never been to an ordinary meeting of doctors when this has ever been discussed, but all the homeopathic meetings I have been to have included doctors from all over the world, and veterinarians. The vets say that doctors have the easy job because they only have to deal with one animal and vets get all the rest. The only difference is that most humans can talk.

The UK ranks at the bottom of the list for treating common cancers. Where Japan is number one, the UK ranks 30/32 for lung cancer and 23/32 for prostate, breast and bowel cancer.

We sow the seeds of our own destruction. The desire for good health and long life pushes us to invent more invasive and powerful technologies, but these may be destructive. X-rays and scans help diagnoses, but repeated X-rays and scans, e.g., mammograms, can cause cancer. The rest of Europe uses proton therapy for cancer treatment. Proton beam treatment is available in four hospitals in the UK but it is not available for all cancers as it is in Europe. It gives better results as it is a more concentrated beam which targets the cancer and causes less damage to surrounding tissue. Is it all due to money?

Could your doctor have unknowingly caused your bowel cancer? Antibiotics may be lifesavers for sepsis and other serious infections, but they wreck your microbiome and a disordered biome (dysbiosis) is what causes bowel cancer.

Life Expectancy

Life expectancy has been rising for more than 30 years – until now. Data shows that what was assumed to be an inexorable rise has been reversed. It also shows that some babies born today will live longer, but the number of years they can expect to stay in good health is falling. Illness and disability will trouble us for the last 20 years of our lives. Will the NHS and social services cope? These figures cannot project the future, as we now need to take into account the rise of autism, which is untreatable with conventional medicine, diabetes, childhood and teenage cancers, all adult cancers, and dementia.

Chronic Disease

Modern medicine is not good at treating chronic disease of any sort. It never cures, only manages. All chronic disease is more common now. This is one of the reasons for specialisation. It is too difficult for consultants to know about everything. If you have a chronic disease you will undoubtedly end up on long-term medication. As this medication only suppresses your symptoms but does nothing for the underlying causes, it will be unlikely that your condition will get better on its own. You will be faced with years of hospital visits to outpatients and years of trying different medications.

To begin with you might find you get on well with the medication, but after a while you get less help from it. If you are lucky there is something else you can try. If you are unlucky you get immediate side effects. The suggestion then is that another tablet is added to your regime to mop up the side effects of the first one. You are advised to keep persevering as side effects often settle. Sometimes you have to take the medication for a long time before the effects are noticed.

I used to think of the mantra, 'If in doubt, blame the medication', when faced with unexplained symptoms in a patient on medication. There is considerable chronic disease from medication, including addiction. There is even medication for you if you have no proven disease, but might get one. Big pharma would ideally like us all to be on medication for life.

What part does medication play in a healthy old age? Only a small proportion of older people are not on any medication. I have felt for years that when the doctor signs a death certificate there should be space for a list of all the medication the patient was taking. In fact, drugs do not only cause side effects but can actually induce problems like hearing loss. It is well known that loud noise damages the nerve to the brain from the ear, but not so well known that aminoglycosides and other antibiotics, platinum-based chemotherapy, salicylates, non-steroidal anti-inflammatories like ibuprofen, loop diuretics and vaccines, to name but a few, can also cause deafness.

Is it time we saw the bigger picture and put the art as well as the science back into healing?

A patient went to see a consultant privately. She paid a lot of money for a 20-minute consultation. As he was ushering her out of the room, she turned to him and asked: 'Tell me doctor, what has caused my problem?' He very patronisingly put his arm round her shoulder and patted her. 'My dear,' he said. 'We don't do causes.' That about sums it up. If you don't do causes, how can you put it right?

Modern Medicine

1. Provides the name of the condition you have, if you are lucky.

2. Provides medication, in terms of antihypertensives, histamines, biotics, epileptics, coagulants, etc. Hence suppression of symptoms, not cure. I asked the medical students what symptoms were. If they reflected the body's attempts to heal, is it right to suppress them? The body's efforts should surely be encouraged and not eliminated. The symptoms are trying to tell you something. Pain on movement suggests the patient should remain still. Exhaustion suggests the need for rest – physical and mental.

3. Never looks for a cause – or it says something vague like 'autoimmune', without explaining why this is happening to you, because it is not known.

4. Provides side effects to medication – mild, moderate or severe, including death. I saw two patients who had developed fibrosing alveolitis of the lung whilst taking atorvastatin. This condition is listed as a side effect of this medication and is irreversible even if diagnosed and the medication halted. The GPs, who did not recognise the disease as a side effect to the medication, were reluctant to stop it for one patient who had had a heart attack. The wife of the other patient said to me that it was logical that if you want to lower the cholesterol levels that cholesterol had to come from some part of the body. Yet the body is full of cholesterol in lots of different organs like the brain, skin and lungs. It is also needed for healing and reducing inflammation. If you take cholesterol out of the lungs the alveoli shrivel and scar. This is exactly what her husband had, but in his case, it was called fibrosing alveolitis, meaning scarring and inflamed alveoli in the lungs. None of their GPs or consultants thought the condition might have been side effects of the medication, although I did find it in the list of side effects online.

5. Provides good emergency care – from paramedics, the fire service, and the army war-zone first aid for treatment of injuries. All this filters down to A & E. But there is no medication to treat shock, hence post-traumatic stress

disorder (PTSD) is common, especially in patients who have been in intensive care. A & Es in other countries, where the homeopathic remedies aconite (for shock) and arnica (for injuries) have been given, report that their patients recover more quickly with less consequent mental health problems. What a lot of money and need for psychological services that would save. It is easy to give homeopathic remedies to unconscious patients as they are absorbed from the buccal mucosa and can be administered as a fine powder or liquid drops.

6. Provides diagnoses by negatives. Going to the doctor with a written list of symptoms to help you remember is a good idea, but your doctor looks at the list and cannot see a pattern, so he says he can only look at one symptom at a time, suggesting he cannot cope, and so sends you for blood tests. He says if you have not heard in a week he has not found any abnormalities. After an anxious week waiting to hear, nothing is heard, which means that your tests were normal. However, you still have the same symptoms and feel most unwell. The next doctor you see, because the first doctor is not available, says he will repeat some of the tests just to make sure that nothing has changed since the last tests, but he too does not know

what is wrong. You are bewildered. How can you have something the doctors cannot identify?

The next doctor this particular patient sees is me and she shows me her original list. Can I tell her what is wrong? The list shows symptoms of anxiety and I tell her so. 'I thought so,' she says, 'but why could the other doctors not identify the problem?' The extra training I have had in homeopathy enables me to identify patterns of disease and so I recognise hers. It is such a waste of time and money sending patients for unnecessary tests when the doctor has no idea of the diagnosis. It would be better to train doctors more thoroughly.

Doctors do not seem to think beyond the obvious to work out what might be causing the patterns they see before them, because they are not taught to put systems together, only to see patients with disease in one system. If a patient attends with backache, how often do 'top specialists' look at posture and see if one leg is shorter that the other? If you do Alexander training or yoga you will learn about the relevance of posture and muscle tension. Then a whole new range of diagnostic possibilities opens up and the doctor should be able to advise the patient accordingly. This can be particularly with regard to some seemingly unusual symptoms, as in fibromyalgia syndrome, when the symptoms are not always in one place and may move around.

7. Means treatment is underpinned by data, or should be. Outcomes of interventions, which are what every patient wants to know, are often unavailable or inaccurate and may depend on the skills and knowledge of the individual doctor. Specialists have meetings and will discuss their treatments, all deciding the best way to treat this particular variation, say, of breast cancer. They never discuss why the patient has this particular problem at this stage in her life. They do not think it is relevant.

One in four patients who have back surgery claim to have been damaged, i.e., they feel worse than they did before the surgery. A mandatory database of surgery for backs will now be kept to see what problems arise. Consultants will be stopped doing operations privately as insurers will no longer pay. The problems seem to be as a result of mistakes.

8. Suggests surgery may remove what is on the surface of the disease, for example a lump, but does not remove (cure) the mechanism that caused the lump originally. Cure may be inadvertent, for example, appendicitis,

where the removal of the appendix will allow the patient's own healing systems to mop up any problems. In fact, the same applies to any condition that antibiotics are given for. The antibiotics kill the germs and the body does the curing.

There have been a number of outcome studies done from the homeopathic hospitals in Britain for chronic diseases, and usually the average outcome score is 75% improvement. It is rare to have patients who are worse on follow-up. This is a very interesting pattern in view of the fact that most people who seek homeopathic treatment have been everywhere, seen every specialist, tried every treatment, had many side effects, and have made no progress. We call it the TEETH syndrome, which stands for 'tried everything, even try homeopathy'. Of course, people who have a terminal illness have a poor prognosis, although there are reported cases of patients doing very well with homeopathy. I had a patient who had a prognosis of six weeks for her pancreatic cancer, who survived eighteen months, and a young man with bladder cancer regrowth whose cancer disappeared.

9. Provides an online record of all the side effects for every medication prescribable. If it were in book form, as

it used to be, it would run to 1,500 pages. There are no side effects with homeopathy, other than the occasional aggravation. This usually occurs with people who have an allergic disposition, and once the aggravation settles of its own accord the patient is considerably better.

Common conventional medication for which I often had to look up side effects were warfarin, statins, aspirin, allopurinol for gout, which seems to also be much more common now, metoprolol, and pantoprazole. Conventional medicine makes many claims for its efficacy, but in 50% of 3,000 drugs there was no evidence of efficacy for them. America's drug watchdog recommended halving the dose of a frequently prescribed sleeping tablet for women. Researchers have discovered that the female body, for unknown reasons, does not metabolise drugs in the same way as men, which meant that as the drug manufacturers had not tested it in women, they were not aware of this fact. Women are slower to break down a drug's active ingredients. Men and women react differently to illness; for example, when having a heart attack, a man clutches his chest because of the severe pain which radiates down his arm. In 20% of women, however, symptoms build up slowly and appear more generalised. Consequently, women seek help less quickly and are more likely to be sent home undiagnosed.

The medical establishment was built by men, uses tests designed for men, trials its drugs on men, and treats men as the default human. Men react to pain differently and are thought to be more stoic and therefore more likely to be treated with analgesics. Boys don't cry. However, male sufferers of breast cancer and osteoporosis may get a poor deal because of its relative rarity. A lady of 60 fractured her wrist in four places. She asked the doctor who looked at her X-ray in the clinic if there was osteoporosis present. He looked at her and said, 'all elderly ladies have osteoporosis'. She felt belittled and categorised (as elderly), ignorant, and definitely a second-class citizen.

I used to ask the medical students I taught to find a definition of 'cure', and to write a list of all conditions cured by modern medicine. The definition that we arrived at, was that all symptoms had gone, no new ones had been produced, no organs were damaged in the process, and medication was no longer needed, i.e., the person was restored to full health without the need to keep taking medication. Using this definition, they were only able to find a few examples from conventional medicine. The usual one was surgery for appendicitis, replacement of joints, and the occasional serious injury. No chronic disease fulfilled the criteria.

Problems around Fertility and Childbirth

Fertility problems are much more common now. Women are often told that they are not ovulating, or the man is having trouble with a low sperm count. The diagnosis of non-ovulation is not a cause. Something must be preventing it. If the man's sperm count is normal it is the woman who is investigated. If the man's sperm count is abnormal it seems to be very difficult to find the cause, and usually no attempt is made.

A common problem now is endometriosis. I have seen this condition increase from rare to frequent. It is diagnosed after an endoscopy and the patient is offered medication, usually an oral contraceptive, which stops ovulation. The thought process was that if there is no ovulation there would be no menses, therefore no retrograde menstruation. If the patient wanted to become pregnant, however, this was obviously the wrong thing for them to do.

I did a study of a number of patients who had been treated with homeopathy and discovered that the problems seemed to stem from retrograde menstruation which was not absorbed once it was in the peritoneal cavity. In healthy women retrograde (back down the fallopian tubes) menstruation is normal, and the endometrium is reabsorbed with no difficulties. If you biopsy the peritoneum in women having surgery for other reasons you find endometrium in various stages of absorption. So, the fault seems to be in the immune system of the peritoneum. What causes this fault? I discovered that all the women had had lots of antibiotics for infections such as acne, recurrent tonsillitis and cystitis. Their gut biome was wrecked and this caused the problem in their immune system in the peritoneum. It was another inadvertent iatrogenic disease. The whole situation was aggravated by a high-sugar diet, usually from anxiety about the endometriosis, and recurrent vaginal thrush was the norm, thrush being an outward sign of dysbiosis.

Endometriosis is a disease where there is endometrium all over the peritoneum. The body tries to heal but the consequence is that the ovaries have such a tough coating that they are unable to release an ovum. The patients who were treated with homeopathy all improved, and some became pregnant.

I also treated women with fertility problems who did not have endometriosis. One lady of 34 had been attending the fertility clinic at the local hospital for seven years. She had been eventually offered IVF, and this had failed. When I took her history there was no illness present and nothing untoward in her past. She had been healthy all her life and was not on any medication. She had not taken antibiotics. I therefore asked about her parents and she said that she had never met her father as he had died just before she was born. I asked from what he had died. The answer was TB. I gave her the homeopathic tuberculosis vaccine (nosode) and she became pregnant on her third cycle after the medication. She went on to have another child three years later. There was no way that modern medicine could have been interested in her father's health or known about the relationship between his health and her infertility problem, or been able to treat it.

IVF involves a lot of difficulties for the woman, who has to have medication to stimulate her ovaries to produce more eggs than normal. She then needs surgery to collect the eggs and they need to be incubated with sperm cells.

The resulting developing foetus is checked for abnormalities and then put back into the uterus. The question then is whether or not the process will succeed. If the cause of the infertility has not been established, at its deepest level, the whole process is extremely risky. The outcomes from IVF are therefore poor. Paying to become a private patient, you might easily be asked to pay for add-ons which supposedly improve the outcomes. However, these add-ons often have no proven effects. There is an increased risk of miscarriage, especially if more than one foetus is put in. No one I have treated has ever been tested for viruses in the endometrium.

The miscarriage and stillbirth rate is also increasing. The definition of a stillbirth is a foetus born dead after 24 weeks of gestation. Before then it is a miscarriage. The risks include smoking, diabetes, and a big group defined as 'unexplained'. Nearer-to-term premature births can occur when there are multiple pregnancies, often as a result of IVF. There are 3,600 premature births per year, which is 1 in 200 births and is equivalent to the total birth rate for one maternity unit per year.

Birth Defects

Ten per cent of children now have a birth defect and in some there are placental complications with poor function. Other problems are pre-eclamptic toxaemia, cord round the neck, infections, obstetric cholestasis (jaundice), and maternal infections with bacteria like streptococci, E. coli, klebsiella, enterococcus, haemophilus influenza, chlamydia, and mycoplasma. Viruses which damage the foetus are rubella, influenza (so never have the flu vaccine when pregnant), parvovirus, coxsackie, cytomegalovirus, herpes simplex, listeriosis, leptospirosis, Lyme disease, Q fever from farm animals, toxoplasma, and malaria. The Zika virus in South America causes anencephaly. Why is there no research into which virus may have caused your child's birth defect, or what may have caused other developmental abnormalities, like cleft palates or Down's syndrome? Infectious agents could easily switch genes on or off which would cause abnormalities. Medical drugs like thalidomide caused problems with limb development, and some anti-epileptic drugs can also cause problems with developing foetuses.

Extra risks include multiple pregnancies, a baby that is small for dates, a mother who is over 35, smoking, alcohol, drugs (both recreational and medical), obesity, diabetes, and epilepsy.

Other Birth Defects

One in fifty babies is affected by birth defects, which is double the number 30 years ago. What is the role of nutrition in this problem? Genetic and chromosomal defects account for children born with Down's syndrome, congenital heart disease and neural tube defects like spina bifida. In Iceland, all patients with Down's syndrome pregnancies are offered terminations. The aim is to rid Iceland of people with Down's syndrome. In this country, when Down's syndrome is identified, termination is offered and 43% of patients take it up. However, there are still the same number of children born with Down's syndrome as there used to be 50 years ago, which means that there would now be double the number of children alive if termination of pregnancy had not been offered. What causes the extra chromosome to occur? Who does any research? The extra chromosome seems to be random, but everything must have a cause. A nutritional researcher

I once talked to said that he thought Down's syndrome was caused by a low level of selenium in the fallopian tubes, which aged the ovum on its way down. I found this very interesting as there is no natural selenium in the soil in the UK.

Risks at the Time of Birth

Birth is one of the riskiest things in the whole of life. It is also one of the commonest times for patients to make complaints afterwards. Usually the complaint involves poor decision-making on behalf of midwives and doctors. There is such a lot that can go wrong. Why are so many babies born prematurely? Why do women often go into labour so early? A very low birth weight baby is at considerable risk of severe learning difficulties and physical problems. Babies born naturally pick up their biome from their mother's vagina. Babies born by caesarean section only pick up skin bacteria so have a poor biome, and consequently are at risk of infections. Does anyone know if babies born by caesarean section are more at risk from autism or sudden infant death syndrome?

The worst possible outcome is that the mother then develops a breast abscess when trying to breastfeed, and is put on antibiotics, which wrecks her biome and that of the baby. The baby also suffers from shock at this time (foetal distress), and as there is no medical treatment for shock, the outcome might easily be poor. Hopefully the baby does not need a vitamin K injection at birth, as this contains alcohol and the neonatal liver is unable to process alcohol. Jaundice may then occur. Despite patients' medical histories and family histories as indicators, it is most unwise to give newborn babies vaccines. Their immune system is not sufficiently developed to cope.

Risks in the Neonatal Period: Low Apgar Score

The Apgar score is a way of assessing the health of babies at birth. An Apgar score of ten represents the best possible condition – meaning a fit and healthy baby from the point of view of its breathing, muscle tone, heart rate, skin colour, and response to stimulation. There should always be concern for a baby that is born with a low Apgar score, and the baby should be followed up by developmental paediatricians. Hopefully the baby will be breastfed and will develop a normal biome.

The next thing the baby has to contend with is vaccination.

Vaccination

The NHS has a routine immunisation schedule that starts at 8 weeks of age. At this point the baby is given DTP (diphtheria, tetanus and pertussis – the latter more commonly known as whooping cough), and polio, haemophilus influenzae B (Hib), pneumococcus, meningococcus B, and rotavirus.

After a period of four weeks' recovery, at 12 weeks, DTP, polio, Hib, and rotavirus are given again.

People only need tetanus protection if they are going to work in certain jobs, such as farming. I saw tetanus in neonates when I worked in Nigeria, because the village people believed the cord remnants should be dressed with cow dung to prevent bad spirits from invading the baby. There was one case in our area of the UK in a lady who put horse manure on her roses and pricked her finger.

However, that was 40 years ago. She recovered. There were seven cases in the UK in 2013 and due to advances in intensive care, none died, so why still include it in the vaccination schedule when the risk is so low? It is always given when people have had a road accident, but that dates to the pre-World-War-I era when there were horses pulling carts on the roads.

In 2016 there were more than 5,000 cases of mumps in vaccinated people and 19 outbreaks on college campuses. So, were some people unvaccinated or had the protection worn off? Or had it never developed in the first place? Is it checked out?

The one vaccine missing is for the streptococcus which causes scarlet fever. None has ever been developed. There are still epidemics occurring but the disease is much milder than it used to be in Victorian times when countless children died. It is now treated with penicillin. There are still consequences from the streptococcus. Recurrent tonsillitis can lead to Tourette's syndrome when the streptococcal toxin is deposited in the brain. Penicillin has no effect on the toxins secreted by the bacteria, only on the bacteria itself.

At 16 weeks, a baby gets even more vaccines: DTP, polio, haemophilus influenzae B, pneumococcus, and meningitis B. Then, at one year of age – Hib plus MenC, pneumococcus, MMR and MenB. It always seems strange to me that MMR is not given until one year of age. Measles was cited as a killer of babies under a year old. It was used as a strong argument for babies having immunisations. It seems as if the other illnesses like diphtheria were much more threatening than measles, and the vaccine for diphtheria was therefore given at a younger age. Measles were common, but death and handicap as a result were rare.

2 to 7 years old: Annual injection of influenza, because flu has a higher mortality rate in young children.

3 years and 4 months old: DPT, polio and MMR.

Girls aged 12 to 13: Human papillomavirus is given in two doses, 6 to 24 months apart. This is given to prevent cancer of the cervix, a sexually transmitted disease. There are alarming reports of illness and death in vaccinated girls from the USA, and two new syndromes have been described in girls who have had this vaccine. CRPS, or Complex Regional Pain Syndrome, when the sufferer has widespread pain, the cause of which cannot be identified, and POTS, Postural Orthostatic Tachycardia Syndrome, which describes rapid heartbeats on change of posture.

14 years old: DPT, Meningitis A, C, W and Y.

Travel Vaccines: Travel abroad, particularly to tropical countries, can be lethal, and vaccines are advised for hepatitis A and B, cholera, typhoid, yellow fever, rabies, encephalitis, meningitis, and medication for malaria. Some countries will not admit you unless you have been immunised.

65 years old: Pneumococcus and annual doses of influenza are given in September/October. This always seems strange to me to offer influenza in September, when it is not a long-lasting protection and most flu does not occur until February or March, by which time the vaccine effect will have worn off.

70 years old: Shingles vaccine is available (Herpes Zoster).

I am concerned that GP practices get paid for their nurses to do the immunisations. This suggests that not only are medical staff not taught about the overuse of conventional medical treatments, but they are given profit-driven incentives to use and overuse more of them. Big pharma makes sure that everyone gets their vaccines.

If you decide to have vaccinations, consider asking the nurse about what is in them. Ask to look at the inset with the ingredients list. They contain altered virus, killed bacteria, formaldehyde, aluminium (toxic to children's brains), possibly mercury, monosodium glutamate, sodium phosphate, phenoxyethanol, gelatine (from animals), sulphites, which people can be allergic to, yeast, antibiotics, RNA and DNA from animal and human (foetus) cell tissue cultures, ethylene glycol (antifreeze), triton (a detergent), and polysorbate, which can also cause allergic reactions. In Finland, they decided that it was better to give vitamin D3, which is safer and makes people 50% less likely to get flu.

For how long are they effective? The flu vaccine may be effective for only a few months, and it may be different in different people. Therefore, if you have the vaccine in October it may be ineffective in March when the flu is epidemic. It may also be ineffective because the vaccine is made from the wrong virus. No information is given for the other vaccines, and it will be different in different people.

What side effects does the vaccine cause? Are side effects recorded? Have they been tested in babies? Or in humans? What financial arrangements are made with doctors to give vaccines?

There are selected immunisation programmes for neonates with hepatitis-B-infected mothers, and infants in areas of the country with TB.

The pneumococcal and flu vaccine are recommended for patients with underlying medical conditions such as splenic dysfunction including sickle cell disease, coeliac disease, cochlear implants, chronic illness such as heart conditions, severe asthma, heart failure, COPD, chronic neurological conditions like Parkinson's, motor neurone disease, learning disability, diabetes, chronic kidney disease, chronic liver conditions, haemophilia, immunosuppressant conditions due to disease or treatment by steroids, immunosuppressant drugs, and chemotherapy. People in residential care or who work in one are also offered the flu vaccine.

There might be a catch-22 situation here, as it is thought that vaccines cause autoimmune disease. When a vaccine is given it may affect the immune system and cause the T-lymphocytes to attack your body. There are more than 80 autoimmune diseases, including type 1 diabetes, Guillan-Barré syndrome, idiopathic thrombocytopenic purpura, narcolepsy, transverse myelitis, multiple sclerosis, rheumatoid arthritis, hepatitis A, lupus erythematosus, Sjorgen's syndrome, coeliac disease, scleroderma and Grave's disease of the thyroid.

There is no doubt that diphtheria, tetanus, whooping cough, polio, mumps, measles and rubella have more or less disappeared from the modern world. However, there is evidence that measles is still about as people can be infected after attending large functions such as outdoor festivals. It is not clear whether the people who develop measles under these circumstances have never been vaccinated or if the effect of the vaccine has worn off or the virus has mutated in some way. It is, however, known that vaccinated people can still get measles. The childhood diseases undoubtedly damaged and killed a few children but having the disease would have developed most children's immune systems, something not measurable at the time, and not damaged their T-lymphocytes.

There is growing concern that the number of vaccinations given alters the immune system in such a way that it could make it more likely for people to develop serious chronic diseases. It begs the question whether there's a relationship between the effects of the vaccinations and cancers in childhood or later, mental health issues, onset of neurodegenerative disorders, and other chronic diseases.

The way vaccines were manufactured until recently meant that considerable numbers of children throughout the world got regular doses of mercury. This was used in the vaccine to stabilise it. Mercury, of course, is highly toxic. What damage has that done to the children who were immunised with it? Mercury is known to cause demyelination, and that would pose a problem for the developing brain and nervous system. Will a generation of children be casualties of progress?

Why is juvenile arthritis so common now? On average young people with arthritis visit their GP four times before referral, and there can then be a delay of three months before seeing a consultant. Tens of thousands of young people have arthritis – mainly rheumatoid, psoriatic, and juvenile 'idiopathic arthritis', which means that the doctors have no idea what it actually is. Could it be related to vaccination? If you get an altered virus from a vaccine in your joints what damage does it cause? Whenever an epidemic of rubella occurred there were always a few people who would present with an acute polyarthropathy, which was usually self-limiting. If the rubella vaccine alters the immune response, the ensuing arthritis could be permanent.

Despite having so many different vaccines now, the population is the sickest ever. Have we swapped low levels of infant mortality for huge increases of later-life mortality and morbidity?

Flu Vaccine

The Cochrane Review of flu vaccines in babies, the middle-aged and the elderly showed that it only worked in 10% of people.

The incidence of flu in the community apparently relates to vitamin D levels. A study in Hong Kong of the flu vaccine versus placebo showed that 5.5 times more respiratory infections occurred in the vaccinated group. There was no difference in incidence of flu in both groups. You exchange a minute chance of avoiding flu for a large chance of more severe colds which last longer. Take vitamin D instead.

Do the vaccines interfere with the cell mediated immune response and cause significant increase in disease of other types?

Vaccines were tested on healthy young men before being put on the market, but what if you are not healthy? The flu jab is deliberately given to people with asthma, heart disease, diabetes, etc. The indications for the flu vaccine have now expanded considerably since it was introduced, which means a much wider market for the vaccine.

When vaccines were originally tested in humans, 'effectiveness' meant 'produces antibodies'. Are the antibodies exactly the same as the body would produce if it were invaded by the wild virus? If they are *not* identical does this mean you are protected? If they are *not* identical does it mean they are safe? Does the body respond differently to attenuated viruses?

There are homeopathic vaccines available for every single disease. They are used extensively by the Cuban government to prevent and treat epidemics of Leptospirosis, in Brazil for meningitis, and in India for a number of diseases where there are no other options, like Q fever. They are even used for the prevention of malaria, another disease for which there is no conventional vaccine.

Increasing Incidence of Chronic Disease

There is an increase in incidence of all chronic disease, including diseases never described before. Some new diagnoses have occurred as a result of scans, especially brain scans in dementia which show subdivisions of categories. This seems to bear out the homeopathic principle that your disease is in an individual pattern, but the basic disease is the same.

There is a huge increase in asthma, with 1,000 patients per year dying. One in twelve adults has asthma and it is as common in the countryside as in cities. Four per cent of the world's population has diabetes, which means 143 million people. By 2025 there will be 5.4% of the population affected. There has been a dramatic increase in the incidence of eye disease, especially cataracts, age-related macular degeneration, glaucoma, and diabetic retinopathy, all of which are mostly explained by the number of older people. If the cause of these illnesses were not just put down to age, they would be more easily treated. It is impossible to find any outcome studies for these problems.

A lot of diseases that used to be confined to the elderly are now becoming diseases of younger people. All forms of cancer, dementia, mental health problems, hypertension, heart disease, hypothyroidism, and asthma have all become common in younger people.

Vaccines have never been tested on children, the elderly, people with pre-existing diseases, or during pregnancy, and rarely on women in general.

Pitfalls in Prescribing

One in twenty prescriptions from general practitioners contains an error (GMC, 2012). If there are 900 million prescriptions annually, then there will be 4.5 million errors annually. The errors are usually mild or moderate, but 1.6 million contain a serious error, which could become potentially dangerous. These contain the following:

- Incomplete information, most commonly the dosage strength and incorrect timing of doses, followed by failure to arrange appropriate monitoring;

- Risk that increases with the number of medications prescribed;

- The age of the patient (with children and the over-75s, the prescription is twice as likely to have an error);

- Incorrect types of medicine prescribed;

- Hospital/GP interface (lack of communication).

There are four classes of drugs that are associated with 50% of preventable medication-related hospital admissions. They are:

1. Antithrombotics, especially aspirin, causing mainly bleeding from the gut;

2. Anticoagulants, mainly warfarin, which may cause bleeding from anywhere and interact with many common drugs;

3. Non-steroidal anti-inflammatory drugs, such as ibuprofen, indomethacin, etc., which may cause bleeding, especially in the gut;

4. Diuretics, which can lead to abnormal biochemistry, mainly sodium and potassium.

Prescribing errors feature commonly in Medical Defence Union case files as patient complaints. They may also result in legal claims of clinical negligence or GMC action against members.

Common mistakes include giving medication like penicillin to patients who have a history of an allergy. Another is prescribing non-steroidal anti-inflammatory drugs with warfarin, and prescribing allopurinol for gout in patients who have decreased renal function. The administration of corticosteroid creams over many years causes damage to the skin. Benzodiazepines are addictive, especially if prescribed long-term, and there may be allergies that are not discussed. Drugs can be very risky.

People in high-risk groups on repeat prescriptions should be monitored, particularly children, the elderly on multiple drugs, and people with either renal or hepatic impairment. If homeopathic medicines were used, most of this would not occur.

The background to all this is big pharma. However, without big pharma there would be no antibiotics, which have saved many lives since they were introduced to the general population in 1947. However, we are now in a situation where antibiotics are losing their effectiveness and that will be a problem as sepsis is now a big killer in this country. The drug companies feel that they cannot invest the huge amount of money that it will take to develop new antibiotics, so it will be up to others to see if they can come up with any ideas. If homeopathic medicines were used the need for antibiotics would decrease considerably. Homeopathic remedies are used by organic farmers for infections in their animals, for example mastitis in cows.

People with mental health problems have a poor deal from big pharma. The medication that is available is not always helpful and causes a lot of side effects. It never cures. Big pharma likes its illnesses to be reduced to biochemistry levels, so that a chemical can be found to block a metabolic pathway. This is considered to be the cause of the patient's illness. The fact that this is only part of the total seems never to be considered.

AstraZeneca threatened to reduce its £2 billion annual drug research programme unless NHS cost-saving plans were dropped. It would delay introducing new drugs by three years if they are deemed too expensive. These are mostly cancer life-extenders, which they say would be devastating for patients and demoralising for the scientists who work on them. Philosophically, how does it help to extend a life by months when the treatment is so life-sapping?

Spending on all drugs is increasing more than three times faster than the NHS drug budget.

Patients should be encouraged to ask questions such as: 'Do I really need this test, or investigation, or procedure?' The problem then, is that the doctor may not feel that they can diagnose without tests, and even when there is a diagnosis, prescribing medication is the only way they feel they can help. The words 'there is nothing more I can do for you' are soul destroying for the patient. Even if they are not spoken aloud, the inference may still be there. The patient feels abandoned. This is one of the reasons I studied homeopathy. There is always a homeopathic medicine you can find to help. Add in some dietary advice, and the patient learns that the answer to a lot of illness can be in their own hands. This, plus support from the doctor, and no ridicule about a patient's choice of a method that works for them, make an enormous difference.

Advice from the Doctor

How can you tell if what the doctor tells you is accurate? For example:

- Does salt cause raised blood pressure? No, it is not a cause, merely an added problem. Raised BP is caused by anxiety and anger, often suppressed, which causes the small blood vessels to constrict and raises the BP. This is why most medication is aimed at relaxing the blood vessels without taking the reason for their constriction into account. Blood pressure can be reduced by biofeedback, a method involving relaxation, breathing and taking stresses into account, and by homeopathic medicines, which have the same effects of relaxation.

- Is the BMI (body mass index) an accurate measurement of being overweight? In fact, it misdiagnoses tall people as overweight and short people as underweight. Why do we need such a measurement when it is obvious if people are the correct weight?

- Is exercise good for you? Why do people run marathons? It is an enormous stress on the body and people have died during the events. Running stresses many joints and the heart. Does it mean the damage will heal and you will not need joints replacing in later life? Joint replacement is common in footballers, ballet dancers, golfers and others who play a lot of sport. If you overuse your heart by making it beat faster when exercising, as it is not designed to beat so quickly for so long, will there be scarring as a result? Does anyone know?

- What do annual checks do for people? Especially when they are based on useless tests like calculating your BMI. It costs the NHS a lot of money, as practices are paid to do it. It was mainly designed to identify people who needed long-term medication like statins. The idea was that prevention would be better than cure, but all they seem to do is make people anxious. People end up on statins as a result of having their cholesterol checked, despite the fact that they do not reduce your chances of heart attack or stroke in the future by more than 10%. A better measure of risk for heart attacks would be levels of homocysteine, as the levels can be improved with B vitamins, especially B3 (niacin). You may be given drugs for blood pressure without 24-hour monitoring, to see if it is just 'white coat anxiety', and may be put on medication for osteoporosis if your height has shrunk. Does anyone know by what percentage people's bone density should increase per annum on medication for osteoporosis? And does it increase?

How Did We Become Overmedicated?

Big pharma is one of the most profitable businesses on Earth. To make such enormous profits, they have medicalised many different conditions. They've encouraged psychiatrists to identify 265 conditions that could need medication, and a book called the *Diagnostic and Statistical Manual of Mental Disorders III* (*DSM-3*, 1980) was written.

Each time a version of the book is updated, it contains more diagnoses and has caused a paradigm shift in the diagnosis of mental illness. It contains diagnoses of sexual dysmorphia in children, for example. A label is comforting to the patient because he knows he is not the only person with this complaint, and if the doctor can give it a name he obviously knows about it.

However, it has allowed big pharma to design many different medications for these problems, often as a result of molecular roulette. They have peddled the illnesses to persuade doctors to prescribe medication to sell the drugs.

Business deals shape our lives. They are made behind closed doors and deliberately make us think in different ways.

Pfizer, the manufacturer of the drug sertraline, an antidepressant, wanted to bring research and marketing closer together. They devised a tool for doctors to enable them to diagnose depression more easily. A questionnaire was developed for patients to fill in with nine questions about how they had been feeling over the previous two weeks. The doctors diagnosed depression considerably more often than they would have done without it.

The NHS spends £44 million per year on antidepressants and £15 million on benzodiazepines. People get left on drugs because they are not often followed up, as doctors think that depression is an ongoing problem which may not resolve and that people will just stop the medication when they feel better.

ADHD was added to DSM-4 and has caused a huge increase in diagnoses. It is now over-diagnosed and over-medicated, and children with immature brains are given drugs for it, the effects of which – long-term – are not known.

Cholesterol

Statistically, if your cholesterol is raised you are more likely to have heart attacks, vascular disease or strokes. If your cholesterol is raised you will be asked to take a statin. If, however, you ask your doctor why your cholesterol might be raised he will be unable to tell you.

Cholesterol is made in the liver and is a component of cell membranes and of bile for digestion. It is a natural emulsifier. It regulates immunity and defence mechanisms so it is needed for inflammation. It transports lipids across the body and protects veins, arteries and muscles from damage. It maintains the structure of cells and prevents crystallisation of fatty acids.

It provides optimal temperatures to maintain the desired movability of membranes, especially in the lungs, which is why the disease sclerosing alveolitis is a potential side effect of statins.

Cholesterol is involved in the synthesis of neurotransmitters, the nerve impulses through neurons in the brain and nervous system. It has a role in the secretion of enzymes and hormones like aldosterone, oestrogen, cortisone, progesterone and testosterone.

Cholesterol is part of the synthesis of vitamin D3 and therefore in bone calcification and keeps the skin supple and moveable.

If your level is raised should you not ask why? What is my body doing that involves extra production of cholesterol, and is it extra for my needs? Do not tell me that statistics say I will have a heart attack as a consequence. How do you know that the level you have just measured is not the correct level for me at this time?

Conclusions

Avoid the doctor. Avoid taking medication. Avoid vaccines. Try to keep fit and healthy through exercise, a good diet, and a happy, peaceful life.

It appears that most conventional medicine is ineffective, dangerous and expensive. It would be a dreadful shame if this era of the NHS becomes known in the future as the age that bankrupted Britain and caused the population to decline into chronic illness.

3

PSYCHO-NEURO-HORMONO-IMMUNOLOGY:
The Subconscious in Disease

I am not a mechanism, an assembly of various sections

And it is not because the mechanism is working wrongly that I am ill

I am ill because of wounds to the soul, to the deep emotional self.

D. H. Lawrence

The Subconscious

The subconscious is the part of the brain that controls the complex machinery of the body. It operates the body automatically and makes hidden decisions.

It controls activities like vision, hearing, movement, assessment of heat and cold, taste and smell. It keeps the organs working and regulates the immune system. It controls biofeedback from the gut, skin, glands, brain and organs. It is psycho-neuro-hormono-immunology.

87

'Psycho' is your thoughts; 'neuro', your brain chemistry; 'hormono', your hormone system; and 'immunology', your immune system. All of them work without you being aware of them, until there are problems and symptoms that arise.

Subconscious processing occurs in the cerebellum at the back of the brain above the spinal cord. Learning, in any sense, hardwires the brain into automatic and energy efficient outcomes. You never forget how to ride a bike, although a lot of neural pathways are involved in the action.

Electrical activity in minute quantities is involved in the transmission of information across the brain and via the nervous system. It also passes signals across cell membranes and between cells.

Sigmund Freud was the first person to study the subconscious and developed a way of looking at people to see what was hidden. Psychologists identify hidden problems that may be responsible for your current problems even though they are not in your conscious mind. It is as if the problems are stored in your hard drive.

The subconscious must therefore be in all parts of the brain.

Dreams come from your subconscious and surface when you are asleep and the conscious part of your mind is not working. They can be frightening enough to wake you.

A man of 54 consulted me about his headaches. He had had no relief from the doctor's prescriptions and all the tests were normal. He took painkillers most days. He was a gardener and loved to be out of doors. I asked how long they had been present and he told me his mother said they had started at the age of four. At two he had a head injury bad enough to seek medical advice and at four he had another. The doctors he had consulted recently did not seem to be interested in his history and just concentrated on the presenting symptoms. In fact, in homeopathic terms it was an example of the 'never well since' syndrome. To look at his subconscious I asked about dreams. He smiled and said he had a lovely recurrent dream when he became a large bird floating above the countryside. I prescribed three tablets of arnica 200C in one day because of the previous injuries, even though they were 50 years ago, followed by natrum sulphuricum 200C, three tablets only. He came back after a month to

89

say he had gradually had fewer headaches and had not had one for a week. This was the longest he had ever been without, and I suggested he take more tablets only if his headaches returned, which they did not. His dreams revealed what was in his subconscious. The desire to float around out of reach so that he was not bothered by anyone.

The subconscious therefore gathers awareness of the world around you. You are attracted to other people and places by the influence of your senses, vision, smell, etc. These experiences from childhood make you into the person you become with your brain wired up accordingly. We are all individual mixtures of all variables.

The brain is usually on autopilot but the unexpected arouses it to ask if the new thing is a threat or an opportunity. It is an arbiter of conflicting emotions but this depends on past experiences and the way the brain is able to learn, which also depends on intelligence. Your thoughts can allow the brain to be a long-term planner, and this will also depend on previous experiences.

Our conscious mind is less important in our lives than the subconscious, so it is easy to see that it can be changed without us being aware of it and cause disease in this way.

We are not aware of disease until symptoms emerge. By then the disease process could have been developing for sometime.

It is easy to see how mental health problems arise from the subconscious as they are primed by experiences and rewire the brain accordingly. The symptoms of anxiety arise as a consequence when they are not dealt with in a mindful way.

Nightmares are a reflection of severe anxiety/shock which has been wired into the subconscious. They then surface when the body and mind is shut down when asleep. Hence the symptoms of PTSD in remembering past dreadful events. Flashbacks relive the event but conscious remembering is suppressed. Fear, anger, anxiety, and the thought *why me?* are the main symptoms. It can be treated with homeopathy.

Dementia also seems to be a disease of the subconscious in that the brain wants to shut down completely. The brain substance slowly disappears as a result of the 'if you don't use it, you lose it' phenomenon. The reason the brain wants to shut down is that life seems too difficult or too painful. It is never an outward expression that is voiced, but is there an underneath in the subconscious? Patients with dementia improve with homeopathy.

Personality

Your subconscious is the essence of your personality. It may be your saviour if the way you have been brought up means that you are not a risk-taker, so you don't exceed the speed limit, for example, or you are polite to people and do not end up in fights, or you realise that education will get you where you want to be. Life is definitely a game of consequences and you may wish, when you get older, that you had made different decisions. However, we are all victims of the times in which we live as a result of inventions and progress. It all depends on how well your subconscious copes and wires your brain.

Psycho-Neuro-Hormono-Immunology

The science of the study of the relationship between the mind and the body has been described as *mens sana in corpore sano* – a healthy mind in a healthy body – and *adapt or die*.

The human body regulates by means of biofeedback systems, for example the pituitary ovarian axis, which controls the menstrual cycle.

No system works in isolation. Thoughts are transmitted by electrical signals which turn the biochemistry of the brain on or off. The feedback systems can then affect the hormone system and the immune system which again feedback around the body. In homeopathy we call this a cascade effect.

Modern investigations allow scientists to study the brain in much greater detail. We know which systems light up in brain scans under a large number of different situations and diseases. Unfortunately, in practice, this does not help the doctor to treat you.

The theory of P-N-H-I has been around since 1865 when Claude Bernard introduced the concept of the 'milieu interior'. Victorian doctors understood the relationship between the brain and the ovaries in women, as premenstrual syndrome was diagnosed in those days. A homeopathic book published in 1912, *Kent's Repertory*, recognises quite a number of symptoms of premenstrual aggravations, showing that the relationship between mind and body was understood.

Reductionism, which means studying smaller and smaller parts of the body, is interesting and tells us about the functioning of the body, especially the cells, but it does not tell us how things function within the totality. It may be of help to the pharmaceutical industry trying to find drugs for different illnesses, but it only means that their efforts will not cure the illness because the underlying problems have not been worked out. In other words, the cause has not been identified.

Following this idea it can be shown that a disease consists of its totality in each individual patient, and that a diagnosis is a list of symptoms which represent only how the disease is expressed in that individual. The pattern of a chronic disease, with its remissions and exacerbations also reflects this. It explains why some people may only ever have one episode of the disease; others will have remissions, some more frequently than others, and why some will go rapidly downhill. For example, everyone with psoriasis knows what triggers a relapse, but the doctor never asks. Even if they did, they may doubt the patient and not know how to handle the information.

It is easy for the doctor to label a patient's illness as psychosomatic, which is usually a derogatory term, and means that he thinks it is self-induced. In other words, he has no idea about it and is not open to any of the patient's ideas.

If, as a doctor, you specialise in rheumatology, you are not going to be interested in the patient's problems that have led up to the suppression of the immune system and the consequent progression of the rheumatoid arthritis. Dr Hahnemann, the founder of homeopathy, said that if you suppress disease, as happens when steroids are prescribed, the disease only emerges stronger later. Palliation is attractive, instantaneous and tempting. Cure will take longer because more attention is paid to the emotions and background of the patient. It is no good treating a seemingly local disease with local treatment because it ignores the underlying problems. In rheumatoid arthritis the local, presenting symptoms can be in the finger joints. They can be treated with analgesics and NSAIDs. This ignores the fact that RA is a whole-body problem. What if the inflammation is caused by lactose intolerance? How is the biome? Does the patient's job or work aggravate it? Is there a family history of RA? What triggered the situation? Are you under long-term stress? What is your body trying to tell us?

Biofeedback is controlled by the autonomic nervous system. As its name implies, it functions automatically and is in two parts, the sympathetic and the parasympathetic. They work in conjunction to control bodily functions which are not consciously directed, such as breathing, heartbeat, and so forth. The sympathetic part of the system controls the fight or flight effect. The parasympathetic controls mostly digestion, and rest and functions whilst we are asleep. Diseases of the autonomic nervous system are mostly those of insufficiency and occur in peripheral neuropathy, ageing, Parkinson's disease, spinal-cord disorders and some drugs, like beta-blockers affect it.

The autonomic nervous system controls:

- blood pressure, heart, and breathing rate;

- body temperature;

- digestion, metabolism, and therefore weight;

- balance of water and electrolytes;

- the production of bodily fluids including saliva, sweat, and tears;

- urination;

- defaecation;

- sexual response.

It has feedback from every part of the body.

The parasympathetic and sympathetic systems work in conjunction with each other for balance.

The fight or flight reaction is a very important one because it usually takes place as a result of anxiety. If the anxiety is sudden and acute, there is shock and the heart and breathing rates speed up and the body is ready to run away. Therefore, it is easily easy to understand how palpitations arise as a result of anxiety. Palpitations are a sensation from the heart beating more quickly than normal. When people get physical symptoms with anxiety, such as palpitations, sweating or difficulty breathing, they do not always see the connection between their fear and the physical symptoms. This is how panic attacks occur.

The knock on effect of continuous overactivity of the autonomic nervous system will be underactivity of the thyroid gland, Addison's disease (which is underactivity of the adrenal glands), exhaustion, and underactivity of the ovaries with possible infertility. In other words, the target glands are worn out by constant activity from anxiety.

The discipline of P-N-H-I is directly responsible for all endocrine disorders like myxoedema, gynaecological problems including infertility and virtually every other disease, other than those which are strictly genetic, and all of it is subconscious.

Everything is connected to everything else.

Patients rarely know about P-N-H-I, but if they ask the doctor what has caused their problem, the question the doctor should ask the patient is, 'what do *you* think has made you ill?' The patient usually knows, and might then ask if the difficult event that they have experienced, for example, is likely to be the cause. If the doctor then says they have no idea, the patient will be confused. The cause of all illness must come from within. It will not be true if the doctor tries to reassure the patient by telling them it is not their fault that they have the disease, and they should explain to the patient that all disease is generated from inside the body, even if it is an infection like flu. When there is a flu epidemic only a few people go down with it; some have it very mildly, some very badly, some can die from it, and in some it triggers post-viral fatigue syndrome. It all depends on the state of your immune system, and this depends on your state of mind as well as the state of your micro nutrients, like vitamin D.

'Psycho-'
Your Thoughts from the Subconscious

As we will see in the next chapter there is hardly anyone who can live all their life without anxiety. Anxiety pervades everything we do on a daily basis. It is therefore no wonder that from time to time the level of anxiety can escalate putting stress on the immune system. I used to see a regular number of schoolteachers at the end of term or in the school holidays, or even weekends, with problems that had occurred as a result of stress. The body can bear up when it has to, but when the pressure stops the illness occurs.

Thoughts also make us who we are. They have been conditioned ever since we were in the womb. We should be very concerned about the number of young people who have a chronic illness. It seems to suggest that how they are brought up, or conditioned, is not having the outcome that their parents would wish. Psychologists are giving serious thought to what is going wrong and how it can be put right. It is obvious that when children have had a violent upbringing it changes their way of looking at life. Bullying can have exactly the same outcome. The effects of early experiences on children seem to result in cancers, chronic disease and mental health problems. There is also an increase in sudden infant and teenage death syndromes. In the USA the timing of SIDs has been noted to be between two days and two weeks after vaccination.

'Neuro-'
Your Brain Chemistry and Wiring

The brain is the most important organ, and governs the function of everything else in the body. It operates by feedback systems, using both biochemistry and electrical activity and is often likened to a computer. To do this it needs raw materials in the form of good nutrition. Characteristics of the brain's ability to cope is related to IQ and is laid down genetically, but can be developed with good conditioning and education. If the circuits of the brain are overused, various parts run out of raw materials, as in Parkinson's disease, but if they are underused, then atrophy of the brain occurs, as in dementia.

Underuse

'If you don't use it you lose it.' Atrophy of the whole brain can be caused by injuries, infections like encephalitis, drugs (especially recreational), and problems with the circulation of the brain, such as strokes, dementia, learning disabilities, and shrinkage, which occurs naturally with age.

At one time it was thought that the brain would never heal itself if damaged, but scans show that the brain can rewire itself; the better the nutritional status, the better the healing.

Overuse

This means the damaged area runs out of nutrients to heal, resulting in atrophy and diseases like Parkinson's, when dopamine is lost from a small area called the substantia nigra due to death of the cells. When the body's healing mechanism tries to heal the damaged area, scarring occurs and function does not return. This cycle depends on how well both nutritional status and the immune system function.

Hormones

Glands depend upon chemical and electrical signalling to function.

Pineal Gland

This small gland is located at the centre of the brain between the two hemispheres. It produces melatonin, which is derived from serotonin. Melatonin regulates sleep patterns and the body clock.

The pineal gland influences the pituitary gland's secretion of the follicle-stimulating hormone and luteinising hormones, both of which govern the menstrual cycle. It also may govern the actions of recreational drugs and antidepressants like fluoxetine. It has an action on bone metabolism and bone density.

Damage to the pineal gland in children by calcification causes accelerated development of sexual maturity, now more common, as girls as young as nine are menstruating.

Calcium, phosphorus and fluoride deposits in the pineal correlate with ageing and maybe why older people do not sleep as well because less melatonin is produced.

Pituitary Gland

The pituitary controls all the other glands because it secretes hormones that activate or shut them down. The main hormones secreted are the growth hormone, gonadotrophins (which affect the testes and ovaries), and the antidiuretic hormone, which stops the body losing too much fluid, and regulates thirst and hydration.

Underactivity of the pituitary gland in childhood causes dwarfism and in adult women causes amenorrhoea. Overactivity causes gigantism in childhood and acromegaly in adults. Acromegaly is easy to spot in adults because the facial shape changes and hands and feet grow bigger.

The pituitary also secretes the follicle-stimulating hormone, which regulates the menstrual cycle, the thyroid-stimulating hormone, which regulates the thyroid gland, and the adrenocorticotrophic hormone (ACTH), which stimulates the adrenal glands. This hormone is suppressed when steroid medication is taken, whether orally, by inhalation, or by application to the skin.

Thyroid Gland

The thyroid gland sits on either side of the midline of the neck just above the clavicle. It secretes thyroxine which contains iodine. The physiological effects of thyroid hormones are widespread affecting growth, sexual maturation and mental development. Thyroxine also affects metabolism, cardiac output and rate, increased peripheral utilisation of glucose and the conversion of liver glycogen to glucose.

Overactivity (hyperthyroidism) causes a rapid pulse, anxiety, muscle-wasting and weakness with increased excretion of nitrogen, phosphorus and potassium. It is difficult to treat and usually the patient is prescribed beta blockers to control symptoms whilst the body heals itself.

Underactivity, myxoedema raises the serum cholesterol level. Hypothyroidism is common in people with Down's syndrome and now very common in normal adults. Deficiency of thyroid hormones causes tiredness, lethargy, constipation, intolerance of cold, stiffness, aching in the muscles, weakness and tingling in the hands, deafness, menstrual irregularities, and slow pulse rate. It causes facial fluid retention, the skin feels dry and coarse and sweating is absent. Body hair is sparse and short. The voice is croaky and speech slurred, memory is poor and thinking is slowed down. It is treated with an artificial thyroid hormone replacement. Everyone with dementia should have their thyroid gland function checked.

Parathyriod Glands

These are small glands situated in the back layers of the thyroid glands. Their function is to regulate phosphorus and calcium metabolism. Underactivity causes increase in phosphorus and decrease in calcium levels which causes cramps and spasms, cataracts, coarse and dry skin, falling hair, and brittle and deformed nails. It can also cause tetany which is severe, prolonged cramps and muscle spasms. Overactivity of the gland causes a decrease in phosphorus levels and an increase in calcium levels, which causes renal calculus and affects bone metabolism.

Adrenal Glands

The adrenal glands sit on the upper surface of the kidneys. There are two parts to them – the outer cortex and inner medulla. The cortex secretes steroid hormones, mineralocorticoids and glucocorticoids. The steroid hormones are androgens, progesterone and oestrogen. The mineralocorticoids, mainly aldosterone, reabsorb sodium in the kidneys and promote the excretion of potassium. An increased secretion of this hormone can occur in patients with oedema.

Decreased secretion occurs in Addison's disease. As the adrenal hormones regulate plasma volume, blood pressure and the intracellular concentrations of sodium and potassium then the lack of them causes severe illness. Addison's disease is acute adrenal insufficiency and can be life-threatening. Chronic lack of secretion of the hormones as a result of life's stresses causes exhaustion.

The secretion of cortisol and glucocorticoids is regulated by adrenocorticotrophin hormones from the pituitary. These hormones are also involved in blood-sugar regulation and glucocorticoids play an important role in modifying the response to infection, traumas, allergies, and stresses of all types – physiological and psychological. They also feed back into the central nervous system. Adrenal crises can be precipitated by physical and emotional stress.

Overactivity causes Cushing's syndrome, which is obesity, hypertension, decreased glucose tolerance, increase in protein metabolism, amenorrhoea, and increased liability to infection.

The Adrenal Medulla:
The Inner Part of the Gland

Overactivity causes excess secretion of adrenaline and noradrenaline, which puts the blood pressure up, causes attacks of sweating and palpitations, nervousness, apprehension, coldness, pallor, angina, pounding in the head, nausea, vomiting, and abdominal pain – the sort of symptoms you would have with a panic attack or during menopause. If a tumour of the adrenal medulla (called a phaeochromocytoma) is causing the symptoms they are constant, and, if as a result of anxiety, intermittent.

Testes

Underactivity causes low levels of testosterone and is called the male menopause. It results in low libido, erectile dysfunction, fatigue, lethargy, muscle weakness, loss of body hair, breast growth, and decreasing size of testicles. Overactivity of the testes causes an increase in testosterone, the male aggression hormone.

Ovaries

Decreased secretion of oestrogen and progesterone happens at the menopause naturally and causes amenorrhoea. Before the menopause it can be caused by the polycystic ovary syndrome. The secretion of oestrogen and progesterone varies with the menstrual cycle. An increase in secretion of hormones will cause irregularity of the timing of the menstrual cycle and variation in the amount of bleeding.

The Immune System

This consists of the thymus gland, spleen, the bone marrow, and the lymphatic system.

Thymus Gland

This is situated in the upper chest behind the sternum, and is the main organ of the lymphatic system. Its primary function is to produce T-lymphocytes, which control the development of cancer cells and increase in response to infections. The gland grows to a maximum size by puberty and then shrinks. It produces thymosins which are hormones that stimulate the production of antibodies, and T-lymphocytes, which are a type of white blood cell. They help fight infections by trapping and destroying abnormal cells. The gland is very active in childhood.

The function of the T-cells is to kill foreign tissue or tissues infected with virus, and produce lymphokines, which are large proteins that regulate other cells of the immune system and to help to enhance the immune response.

Research suggests that 38% to 45% of autistic children have T-cell abnormalities. In other words, their thymus glands are damaged or not functioning properly. Might the abnormality be caused by vaccine damage to the developing thymus? It would explain the frequent infections.

AIDS is the acronym for 'acquired immune deficiency syndrome', caused by the human immune virus, which kills CD4+ T-cells and developing thymocytes in the thymus.

The Spleen

The spleen is an important organ of phagocytosis. Foreign bodies, viruses and bacteria are ingested and dead cells and cell fragments are removed. It makes and recycles platelets, lymphocytes and monocytes. It is a major site of antibody formation. Is it known how the spleen deals with the abnormal viruses found in vaccines?

Medical theory is that if your child is exposed to a weakened version of the disease, they will produce antibodies to that disease, become immune, and never contract the illness. At first glance, this sounds like a solid principle, but it only focuses on one small aspect of the immune system: the antibodies. It fails to look at all the other functions responsible for protecting your child's health. The immune system is also made up of the skin, mucous membranes in the nose and throat, ears and eyes, nasal hairs, saliva, intestines, tonsils, and even the brain.

• The skin acts as a barrier to prevent bacteria entering the body. It also filters out toxins by promoting fever. A fever is the body's way of trying to kill off invaders. Should we therefore give a child paracetamol to bring down their fever, or would we be better off using a homeopathic remedy like aconite, which would stimulate the body to heal itself?

• The nasal hairs prevent foreign particles from travelling up the nose, and the mucous membranes excrete a substance which is anti-bacterial.

• Tonsils help prevent respiratory diseases and illnesses such as polio. Saliva contains substances which destroy and neutralise microbes.

- The spleen and microbiome, among other organs, send nutrition around the body and protect against viral and bacterial invasion.

- The thymus gland produces T-cells, which are antibodies to infection.

- There are various glands (lymph nodes) in the body that drain it of toxins, and bacteria and viruses. For instance, the cervical nodes drain the head, neck and chest.

- The pituitary gland in the brain directs all of these systems, so if the brain goes wrong, so does the immune system. It sends electrical impulses to all areas of the body, stimulating cell re-generation and muscle growth. These electrical impulses also stimulate the thymus gland – the centre of immune function.

Normally, when bacteria or viruses enter the body, antibodies are produced after being primed by the tonsils that there is impending infection. Therefore, if the infection takes hold, there will be white blood cells ready to neutralise the infection. In the case of vaccination, the virus goes straight into the blood, bypassing the normal route into the body via the nose or throat, and with no opportunity for the body to recognise the invader, no extra immune cells are produced to deal with it. With vaccination there is more than one disease present (e.g., measles, mumps, and rubella, all in one), whereas naturally a child would never contract three diseases at the same time. This puts additional strain on the immune system.

Injection of vaccine via this unnatural route can use up 70% of the immune system's resources, instead of the usual 3% to 4% with a wild occurring disease. Because the body has no extra antibodies waiting to counter the vaccine, it can go into overdrive in an attempt to deal with the situation, taking much needed vitamins away from bones and other organs, to use for the production of more antibodies. This lack of vitamins can also cause bruising, retinal bleeding and haemorrhaging, which is why some vaccine-damaged babies have been falsely labelled as 'shaken baby syndrome' cases. It may also account for the increasing incidence of rickets.

It is in this state of dysfunction and chemical overload, maybe from vaccines, pharmaceutical drugs, pollution,

113

junk food, and so on, that our bodies become less able to stay healthy. This could be described as a manmade disease.

The Bone Marrow

The bone marrow's main function is to make red blood cells. This depends on a good supply of iron, folic acid, and vitamin B12. Lack of these nutrients causes anaemia, which can be a shortage, smaller size, or disfigurement of red blood cells. An excess of red blood cells is called polycythaemia and occurs in people short of oxygen through heart or lung disease.

White Blood Cells

1. Neutrophils

Neutrophils are the most common type of white blood cell in the body. They are medium-sized with irregular nuclei and many granules that perform various functions within the cell.

They function by attaching to the walls of blood vessels, blocking the passageway of viruses that try to

114

gain access to the blood through a cut or infectious area. Neutrophils are the first cells to reach an area where a breach in the body has been made. They kill germs by means of a process known as phagocytosis or 'cell-eating'. Besides eating bacteria one by one, they also release a burst of super oxides that have the ability to kill many bacteria at the same time.

2. Lymphocytes

Lymphocytes are small, round cells that have a large nucleus within a small amount of cytoplasm. They have an important function in the immune system, being a major part of the humoral immune system, which is the part that relates to antibody production. Lymphocytes tend to take-up residence in lymphatic tissues, such as the spleen, tonsils, or lymph nodes.

B-lymphocytes make antibodies and this is one of the final steps in disease resistance. When antibodies are made, they prime pathogens for destruction and then make memory cells ready to go into action at any time in the future. The cells will remember a previous infection with a specific pathogen.

3. Monocytes

Monocytes are the largest of the different types of white blood cells. Monocytes are granulocytes, meaning they have few granules in the cytoplasm when seen under the microscope. Monocytes turn into macrophages when they exit the bloodstream.

As macrophages, monocytes do the job of phagocytosis (cell-eating) of any type of dead cell in the body. Because of their large size, they have the ability to digest foreign particles in a wound, unlike other types of white blood cells.

4. Eosinophils

These have large granules that help in cellular functions. Eosinophils are important in allergies and worm infestations. They work by releasing toxins from their granules to kill pathogens. If you have allergies you will have a high eosinophil count.

5. Basophils

Basophils have large granules that perform functions that are not well known. They are very colourful when stained and observed under the microscope, making them easy to identify. They have the ability to secrete natural anticoagulants and antibodies that work against hypersensitivity reactions in the bloodstream. They act immediately as part of the immune system's function against foreign invaders. Basophils contain histamine which dilates the vessels to bring more immune cells to the area of injury.

The consequence of activity of the white cells is inflammation which itself is a healing mechanism. It should therefore not be suppressed with anti-inflammatory medication.

The emerging pattern is that everything is connected to everything else and depends on the other parts of the body responding. If there is failure of response then disease occurs as in myxoedema, infertility, etc., according to which organs are targeted. The proper functioning of this complex system depends on your genetic make-up, your nutritional status, your mental health and the health of your immune system. Anxiety is usually the cause of change in the smooth working of this system.

It seems that subconscious thoughts influence brain chemistry, the immune system and hormones. You need all of these to function well to prevent or make an illness better.

But what thoughts are likely to influence the system and put it out of balance? The answer is in the next chapter dealing with anxiety and shock.

What Affects the Immune System?

The immune system is constantly checking for any invaders like bacteria and viruses. It is also affected by everything that affects our mood. This is a reflection of our characters and natures. It means that everything is connected.

Some things like laughter and happiness affect us positively. Optimism is expressed as 'always look on the bright side', because the opposite view gets us down. We inadvertently use expressions which reflect the way our immune system works. It is easy to see that if you are continually stressed or worried your immune system is affected and it may result in a cold or some other infection. If part of your immune system is engaged with dealing with how you feel another part may not respond as well. At this point genes are involved because you inherit a good or poor response from the immune system and this causes your illness. It may not be an infection you catch, but as the immune system covers any abnormal situation the result will be cancerous changes. These seem to be an everyday occurrence and are dealt with swiftly. Then it depends on how well your immune system is working whether or not this outcome continues and a cancer develops.

Other things that affect the immune system are responses to the home environment, so keep your home neither too clean not too dirty as exposure to germs stimulates the immune system and living in a rural area where exposure to animal bacteria invigorates your biome, because what you breathe in affects the biome. Take your holidays in the country and not in cities.

A high-salt diet, especially from canned food, affects you by reducing immune function. So does too much exercise, which is why Olympic athletes can develop problems like glandular fever. Too much alcohol affects the biome so can be responsible for illnesses other than liver disease. Nicotine from cigarettes and vaping also depresses the immune system.

The younger you are the more underdeveloped the immune system is, and the older you are the more it is worn out.

Chronic stress, loneliness, loss and grief and suppressing the emotions alter immune-system function. This is where homeopathy is so valuable, as there are plenty of medicines to help with these problems, there being none in conventional medicine. It has always been known by homeopathic doctors that these situations are injurious to health. It used to be referred to as 'dying from a broken heart', which has always been scorned by conventional doctors.

4

ANXIETY AS A BASIS FOR DISEASE

I found I was able to relieve people (by hypnosis) not only of pain but of fear. It is strange how many people suffer from it. I don't mean fear of close spaces or fear of heights, but fear of death and what's worse, fear of life. Often, they're people who seem to be in the best of health, prosperous, without any worry and yet they are tortured by their anxieties. I sometimes thought it was the most besetting humour of men, and I asked myself at one time if it was due to some deep animal instinct that man has inherited from that primeval something that first felt the thrill of life.

The Razor's Edge, W. Somerset Maugham, 1944

Definitions of anxiety include one from a dictionary: unease, concern, troubled. I was unable to find a medical definition. My definition is a constant or intermittent state of fear, which can vary in intensity from mild to overwhelming.

Anxiety can be a learned pattern of behaviour, which is why talking therapies and cognitive behavioural therapy can help. It also seems to be innate, in that it can exist from birth which means it must be learnt in the womb and have a genetic aspect. It often happens that if you are a worrier, someone will tell you that you are just like a particular member of your family.

Types of Anxiety

1. Acute: which is sudden onset of severe fear and shock, for example on hearing bad news, the effects of which can be delayed.

2. Intermittent: anxiety that comes and goes and is variable in its intensity.

3. Cumulative: anxiety that builds upon itself and can escalate into panic attacks.

4. Anticipatory: fear of what might happen, often subconscious. There is a very large group of sufferers, but it is not recognised by conventional medicine. This includes agoraphobia, fear of the future, and fear of death, and is often what wakes people earlier than they would

have liked. It is a common cause of diarrhoea in irritable bowel syndrome.

Every person has their own individual coping level, beyond which their coping mechanisms fail and they become ill. The coping mechanism is the load of anxiety that can be tolerated. When the anxiety level exceeds the coping level symptoms occur. The tipping point is different for each person.

Anxiety Levels, Coping Levels, and Illness

The Yerkes-Dodson Law. Two American psychologists said in 1908 that there is an empirical relationship between arousal and performance. Performance increases with mental and physiological arousal but only up to a point. When levels of arousal get too high performance decreases. Different tasks need different levels of arousal for optimal performance, which facilitates concentration, stamina and motivation. Arousal energises, but too much arousal causes stress which affects attention, memory and problem-solving. The more anxious you become the worse you perform. This applies to academic and sporting situations.

Levels of Arousal

At the baseline the person is under-stimulated (bored) or asleep. With more stimulation they may still be bored, but attention and interest increase and they are alert. Next, they are at optimal performance and arousal. When stress is introduced and if strong anxiety occurs, their performance is impaired. At the end of their coping level they are overwhelmed, distressed, dysfunctional, and may panic. The variation in the speed of arousal and its consequences are personal attributes, and reflect genes and upbringing, as well as the learned ability to deal with the levels of anxiety encountered in life.

Timeline Graphs to Illustrate the Onset of Disease:

1. In the first patient there were no problems with her birth, and none at school, university, in relationships, jobs, or with her finances. She learnt good coping skills in childhood and adolescence, and was accepting by nature. There were never any severe, unexpected shocks in her life, and she learnt to be philosophical about most problems. She never married nor had children. She ate a

good diet and most of her relatives lived to a reasonable age. She also lived to a good age (94) without any major health problems.

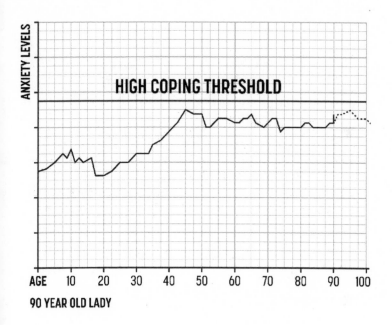

2. The second patient was a male with constant anxiety, a significant life event, and the onset of physical disease. He'd had a difficult birth with foetal distress in labour. He developed normally, and was a happy child until he

was bullied. He was not confident enough to handle it and became increasingly anxious.

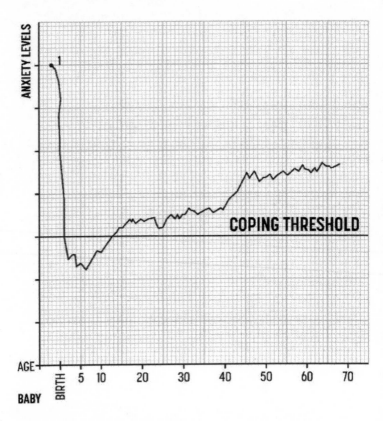

After school he found a job that he liked, but found it difficult to get on with his workmates. He was shy with them, and shy with girls. He was always going down with colds. Eventually he settled down and married, but the strain of looking after a family was too much for him, and his marriage broke up. The divorce was a terrible shock for him. At the age of 50, he developed aggressive prostate cancer, and died at 55.

3. The third patient was a male with severe depression and mental illness. His birth had been normal. He enjoyed school as he was clever. He was never relaxed about relationships, and realised during his teenage years that he was gay. He went to university and became very anxious, as he always wanted to be the best. He was very competitive. At the age of 40 his steady relationship broke down and his anxiety levels increased considerably, until he was in despair. At that point he was diagnosed with depression. However, the medication prescribed did not help, as he started having visual hallucinations. In case the medication was responsible, his GP reduced it slowly and then stopped it. He had no more hallucinations, but was no better. He often felt that life was not worth living and despaired of feeling better. He had spells of CBT (cognitive behavioural therapy), which didn't really help. However, some homeopathic gold – Aurum metallicum – helped him considerably. If he had not had the Aurum, he would probably have been in a state of chronic, severe anxiety for most of the rest of his life.

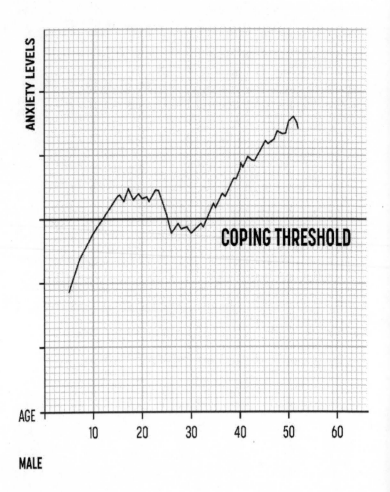

ANXIETY LEVELS

COPING THRESHOLD

AGE

10   20   30   40   50   60

MALE

Anxiety levels vary on a minute to minute basis and are cumulative. If your anxiety does not subside an add-on effect occurs and eventually your level climbs beyond your personal coping level and you become overtly mentally ill. The next stage in the sequence is panic attacks, and when they merge into one another it can turn into mania – plus or minus depression. Then paranoia and auditory or visual hallucinations can occur. If you add despair, sadness, and grief, then suicide is a possibility.

Significant anxiety-provoking events in a person's life may be sudden and profound, or repeated, small, and cumulative. If the significant events are not rationalised by the patient, they become more anxious. People say that you must come to terms with things and just get over them, thinking they are being helpful, but if you are very anxious, you are unable to rationalise.

As with all animals, it is safest to say that all humans are anxious from the foetus onwards, and phobic anxiety states are a protective mechanism to soothe anxieties. As in autistic children their behaviour is a reaction to anxieties they cannot cope with, and putting things in order is a way to soothe them.

Biologically, with anxiety, adrenaline levels are high. As long as nutrition is good enough to support the constant manufacture of adrenaline everything is okay. But if it is not then a shortage produces exhaustion.

Anxiety is measured by psychologists and psychiatrists on various scales, such as the Hamilton Anxiety Rating Scale (HAM-A), and the Spielberger State-Trait Anxiety Inventory (STAI), and sleep disorders on the Jenkins Sleep Scale (JSS). The tests are repeated to see if progress is being made. I find patients' words, mannerisms, and discussions to be more revealing. It seems that if you can't treat a problem, then you should devise a questionnaire to measure and monitor it.

Because anxiety is virtually untreatable other than with tranquillisers – including diazepam (Valium) and chlordiazepoxide (Librium) – and antidepressants (SSRIs, etc.), which are both highly addictive, it is rarely discussed thoroughly with the GP, because in a 10-minute appointment there is simply not enough time to do so. Due to rushed consultations, GPs could have difficulty relating the physical symptoms presented, to a proper diagnosis of anxiety, and thus an effective treatment plan. It is therefore often left to the patient to try to find their own relief for their disorder.

A lifetime of events and anxieties makes you the person you are today, including any physical illnesses you might have had, or currently have.

Low-Level Anxiety

This is mostly anticipatory, with thoughts, for example, such as, *Will I miss the bus? Will I pass the exam? Can I cope with this situation? Will I be bullied today, and what should I do if so?* These common, chronic anxieties can affect your mood (get you down), and may cause gloom or depression. Some people are superstitious and keep good-luck charms and touch them for luck, which gives them confidence. Confidence decreases when people are very anxious.

Stress

Everyone who says they are stressed experiences it in different ways. It may cause insomnia, anxiousness, anger, and give physical symptoms like sweating, poor temperature control, rapid heartbeat, and mood swings. For some, stress is their motivation – until it overburdens them.

Anxiety is the default mode of humans. People who say they do not worry or suffer anxiety usually do not think about it, which means it may be buried in the subconscious. It can surface as dreams when the conscious state is not around to suppress it. Dreams therefore can be very revealing.

If your anxieties stay on the surface and escalate you may get a mental health illness. By that, I mean that you may be ill enough to have a label (diagnosis) given to you. If you suppress your anxieties, you may get a physical illness. Saying your thoughts and problems out loud can lessen the shock, but if you are not used to talking about your emotions, or there is no one to talk to, they get buried.

Anxieties are easy to cope with if you are confident and outgoing, but if you are shy and insecure you may not find ways of helping yourself. One way is anger. Anger arises out of the inability to cope with what is winding you up. Anger is what causes your blood pressure to rise. It has a considerable impact on your physiology.

Trauma from accidents and injuries would appear to be mostly physical, but it can cause severe mental shock. There is no treatment for shock in modern medicine. It used to be hot, sweet tea during the war. The mental aspects of physical injuries are mostly ignored, but can lead to post-traumatic stress disorder. It is now being studied in patients who have been in intensive care units and heavily sedated in order to allow the brain and other organs to heal, and is found to be very common and difficult to treat. It is a pity that the doctors running intensive care units don't know about the homeopathic remedy aconite for shock, as it is used in a lot of hospitals in Europe and India with considerable help to the patient who makes a speedier recovery.

Post-traumatic stress disorder is usually an acute stress reaction, which means severe anxiety was the response to a deeply traumatic situation. You would expect stress to be a natural response, but this state is overwhelming and the victim fails to recover and their mental health deteriorates. It is also treatable with homeopathy.

133

Chronic PTSD can last for many years and can be the result of abusive relationships, particularly in children.

There are reference points in life which help to alleviate anxiety. One is routine. Sticking to the same routine (particularly getting up and going to bed at the same time, eating meals at the same time, and work and play at the same times during the day), trains the body clock to respond in a less anxious way. Routine gives stability.

Your family members can be the making or the breaking of you, according to your relationship with them. Your environment is also important – whether you live in a city with a lot of people and noise, or in the countryside, with fewer people and different types of noise, like birdsong, animals, and tractors. Wherever you live there is traffic of some sort.

Someone who is always in a rush, seems to have too much to do and is always talkative, and rarely quiet and peaceful, reflects someone under stress.

Urbanisation

The vast majority of people live in towns and cities and move around more rapidly than previous generations used to. Walking speeds have risen by 10% since the 1990s. People talk more quickly, act more quickly and are less tolerant of dither and delay. It may be that people who rush around and talk too much wear out the chemicals in parts of the brain, and this is why they get Parkinson's disease. Rushing around and speaking a lot can reflect anxiety.

We like to be excited by information on social media, but being overloaded is stressful. There is pressure to respond. The world is speeding up with big data and faster algorithms. It is a common feeling that time is speeding up. Life seems full of deadlines. It is no wonder that people are exhausted, stressed, and unable to cope. There seems to be no time to stand and stare.

Consequences:

10% of children have mental health problems.

One in twelve adolescents self-harm.

35,000 children are on antidepressants.

30% of children are overweight.

Human beings are now more urbanised. The larger our communities are the faster we move around in them. We easily become harassed and harassment causes loss of memory. If you have just put the washing out and on your way upstairs to see to the bedrooms, you look out of the window and see that it has just started to rain. This distraction make you forget what you went upstairs for. This is a common scenario in menopausal women. It is why people mislay things like car keys. There are too many people, too much traffic, and the pace of life is too fast. This is an overcrowded island. However, relaxation is a state of mind which can be triggered by place and music, and taught in yoga and meditation classes.

The human brain is full of electrochemical signals to connect it up. It decodes the outside world using our senses. It looks at pattern recognition and meaning. Research is showing us how the brain is wired up. There appears to be a zettabyte of information in the human brain. A byte is the unit of digital information and a zettabyte is 10 to the power of 21. How the neurons connect makes a person who they are. The nervous system rewires, reconditions and reconfigures constantly.

Obsessional States

These are unwanted and intrusive thoughts, images and impulses and the resulting behaviour is a way of the brain trying to calm things down. Hoarders, compulsive cleaners as well as people who wash their hands, wash their clothes, tidy up, or always do things in the same order fall into this category. People can be obsessed with celebrities and other people, which may lead to stalking.

Compulsive behaviour is accompanied by feelings of anxiety and the ritual behaviours temporarily neutralise anxiety. If you don't do the obsessive behaviour the anxiety will increase. Swearing is part of an obsessive state.

Somatic States from Anxiety: Or is it All in Your Mind?

These problems used to be called psychosomatic diseases because they could be triggered by anxiety. At one time women who displayed these anxieties were labelled hysterical or neurotic. People who have allergic asthma can have an attack from anxiety when accompanied by hyperventilation.

1. Diseases where there is an observable and identifiable disturbance of bodily functions, as in irritable bowel syndrome, where anticipatory anxiety can cause diarrhoea. Hypertension, tics and spasms, asthma, insomnia, sleep disorders, including nightmares, sleepwalking, bed-wetting, movement problems, sleep apnoea and snoring, psychogenic nausea or vomiting (reflecting the patient trying to say *I'm sick of this!*), difficulty swallowing and eating, skin conditions, and polymyalgia rheumatica, where muscle tension causes pain.

2. Problems where the disturbance is one of perceived symptoms and sensitivity, or excess reaction to normal bodily sensations, like hypochondriasis, which reflects fear of an illness, somatisation disorder, which means that anxieties are translated into physical symptoms like vertigo, dizziness and unsteadiness, and body dysmorphic phobia, when people dislike parts of their body and fear that they are inferior as a result.

3. Problems in which the basis of symptoms varies or is uncertain, like headaches, disproportionate breathlessness, hyperventilation, functional chest pain, and chronic pain.

4. Anxiety produces tension, sometimes called nervous tension, in the muscles and ligaments, which is the field of study of biomechanics: how people's posture results in illness. Curved spine in older people is said to be due to osteoporosis, but as one lady said to me: 'I have the weight of the world on my shoulders and not enough energy to stand up straight.' When we are tired we slump in a chair. We do not stand in the military position any more. No one has deportment lessons. Any spinal or joint pain will be aggravated by tension, and the tendons and ligaments (the hydraulics) will be overstressed and painful. People sometimes don't realise that they jut their chins out, and this puts pressure on their necks, stretches the tendons, and can cause pain. If you have muscular, joint or tendon or ligament pain, learn to stand in the military position, which is called the mountain position in yoga. You may also have one leg longer than the other, and this produces unevenness and strain in the pelvis and gluteal muscles, which could be relieved by a heel lift in the shoe. Tension causes neck pain that disturbs sleep, which causes an immune-system response.

Poor posture and strained ligaments and tendons put unequal forces through joints. So, tension usually causes the hydraulics of the joint rather than the bony structure to be inflamed. Fifty per cent of knee replacements do not cure people's problems. Despite there being osteoarthritis seen on the X-ray it may be the hydraulics that are at fault, and replacing the knee will not help the ligaments.

5. Consequences of long-term anxiety include exhaustion, back problems, walking too fast, speaking too much, being obsessed with detail, being worn out, or an acute or chronic illness that stops you in your tracks and prevents you doing the thing that is causing it. Dementia does this. If you forget, you don't remember you were anxious or in pain.

6. Things to worry about… Money is the main cause for 20% of people. Financial anxiety causes people to be panicky, overwhelmed, disappointed, exhausted, and embarrassed. Financial abuse by a relative or friend can cause severe anxiety. One patient developed delusions that the neighbours were sending offensive messages into her television set, triggered by anxiety about money problems with her son. Banks now have dedicated mental health teams for their customers!

Sigmund Freud thought that anger turned inwards caused depression. People who are angry are also very anxious. If your anxieties overwhelm you and you cannot cope, despair sets in and depression follows. You feel out of your depth, become anxious and cannot cope or make rational decisions.

If you feel safe you are much less anxious. Risk-takers, however, cause themselves anxiety, which causes an adrenaline rush and they can become addicted to that.

Physical Symptoms From Anxiety

Muscle tension, twitching, shaking, tremor, restlessness, easy fatiguability, breathlessness (inability to take a deep breath or hyperventilation) due to tension in the abdominal muscles, palpitations, sweating, dry mouth, dizziness, nausea, diarrhoea, flushes or chills, frequent urination, difficulty swallowing, feeling on edge, difficulty concentrating, insomnia, irritability.

Anxious thoughts include the inability to cope, performance fears, anticipating negative evaluations

141

from others, and diffuse somatic concerns, which is a fear of illness.

Physical symptoms of panic are overwhelming fear or anxiety causing breathlessness, palpitations, chest pain, a choking sensation, dizziness, tingling in the hands and feet, hot and cold flushes, sweating, fainting, trembling, and feelings of unreality (this cannot be happening to me). It doesn't take much to tip a patient – with feelings of unreality and some extra anxiety and fear – over into hallucinations.

There is a scale for every emotion, from virtually none to overwhelming, and we are all somewhere on it. Examples include jealousy and envy, ambition, lustful, glory, making positive choices about how you live, and not letting time drift by, determine your own fate, master of your own destiny, assertive, aggressive, shy, timid, gentle and self-confident. Lack of self-confidence is underneath most mental health problems. Words we use to describe people are extrovert, bold, fraudster, competitive, rivalry, need to win, optimism, exhilaration, enthusiasm, pessimism, and cynicism.

Facts About Anxiety

1. When you are anxious you are uneasy, concerned, troubled, and worried.

2. Fear is an emotion caused by impending danger or evil, a state of alarm, dread of something, anxiety for the safety of someone, afraid of, uneasy anticipation.

3. Worry makes you flustered, full of uneasiness; your face looks anxious or troubled. You give way to anxiety, let the mind dwell on troubles, fret, go over unsolved problems in the mind in a manner which is unlikely to lead to a solution.

4. Sleep is an estate of diminished arousal, but if arousal is increased easy waking occurs, dreams are remembered and early waking occurs.

5. Fear more usually arises from the person's imagination than an actual reality. As a result of fear dopamine is released into the brain and everything becomes a threat. People who have psychotic episodes describe terror, feeling threatened and frightened beyond belief. This can lead to paranoia and hallucinations – both visual and auditory. Antipsychotics, which are major tranquillisers,

reduce the level of dopamine, and the paranoia subsides, but leaves the underlying problem of the causes of anxiety untouched. There is no medication that can rewire the brain and stop the anxiety. Genetics have a small effect, only on psychosis, but the urban environment has a big effect and migration, even if within the country of birth, can also have an effect, as a result of becoming an outsider. The major background is childhood abuse. Life is rarely calm. Cognitive behavioural therapy attempts to rewire the brain, but may take a considerable time. Homeopathic remedies are much quicker.

Stress and anxiety are the major health epidemics of the twenty-first century. They are linked to cancer and heart problems. Millions of people feel close to their breaking point, that is, going above their coping level. They spend a lot of time overbreathing, with an increased pulse rate, changes in body temperature, and exhaustion. If your heart rate is constantly higher than it should be then it does not take much extra stress (plus coffee, for e.g.) to tip it over into irregularity.

When constantly bombarded by stresses like deadlines your blood sugar and cholesterol both increase. If you find out your cholesterol is raised how many doctors ask you about stress? Cholesterol is part of the body's healing mechanism and if it is artificially lowered how does that affect your ability to heal? If your blood sugar is raised, we would say you had diabetes, but how many doctors would ask about stress? Cholesterol and sugar levels can be lowered with medication, which saves having to try to tackle deeper problems. Modern medicine often acts as a mopping up rather than a curing service.

If you also have money worries and things at work go wrong, your body is not coping and you become ill. What you think, you will become. That is, I feel calm versus I feel excited, or I rise to the challenge versus I feel anxious. So your mindset defines your performance.

In chronic stress an increased level of cortisol production is constant. This weakens the immune system, raises the blood pressure and causes heart disease. Anxiety and depression affect lifestyle habits, including eating to try and boost mood when sweet and fat fatty food is craved. Taste is altered by the emotions and we crave comfort food. Treatment that helps in this situation is exercise, tuning it to and managing your stress and mindfulness which is concentrating on what you are doing and not letting your mind wander.

Stress is the external things in our lives that cause anxiety. These include major life changes like births marriages and deaths, moving house, starting a new job, exams and meetings, especially if you are unprepared. You then become overwhelmed and anxious. Symptoms include feeling irritable, fearful, having low self-esteem, indecision, difficulty concentrating, headaches, dizziness, tiredness, appetite changes, being short tempered, having racing thoughts and physical tension. It can also manifest itself as a feeling of uneasiness or sense of impending doom. When anxiety escalates out of control, panic attacks occur. We are overburdening our children and need to remember that half of the population has an IQ of less than 100, the average, and even the people above the 50th percentile will not always cope with academic work. This is why the grammar schools were so successful as they sorted out the children who were likely to benefit from further education. Children now may have difficulty coping because they have undiagnosed problems that rarely existed previously, like dyslexia.

Children are very stressed by their education nowadays. Before the eleven-plus was abolished and children went to grammar schools or secondary moderns, there were hardly any mental health problems among schoolchildren.

146

The grammar school children were pushed educationally, but the children at secondary moderns were taught more practical skills. This suited a lot of them more than having to do GCEs, and caused less stress for them. Nor were they constantly monitored. They just did end of year exams. Teachers knew their pupils and did not get stressed having to produce statistics for the government. Only 3% of children used to go to university, but since the definition of university has widened, 50% of children are pushed to go. A lot of people would prefer to do much more practical training, as it would suit them better and not cause so much anxiety. There were, of course, no computers to alter our lives then.

More than 700 primary schoolchildren were treated for self-harm in London hospitals in 2016. Growing numbers of teenagers are also hurting themselves. There were 729 admissions in London for children of primary school age in 2015–16. Academic worries, cyberbullying, and anxiety about not having enough social media 'likes' were fuelling mental health issues in children as young as eight.

This is obviously very worrying, but suggests that children are not learning to behave in a civilised way towards others. Civilisation... is behaving towards others as you would like them to behave to you.

The consequences of so much stress for children are wide ranging. There has never been so much chronic disease and cancer in people below the age of twenty.

Shock

Stress tends to be chronic, but shock is sudden and deep-acting. The child or family does not have to be aware that there has been a shock, because it may be silent and produced by the subconscious. The brain can receive a shock, suddenly shut down parts of its circuits, then subsequently try to rewire. The consequence is problems in the brain chemistry and the knock-on effect is damage to the hormone and immune system. As we will see in the chapter about autism it can cause severe illness.

A lady of 36 had a sudden, severe shock when her mother was killed in a road accident. Three months later she discovered a lump in her breast that was a cancer. Her surgeon told her that there was no connection between the two events, but she knew differently.

It would appear that we should pay attention to teaching our children how to be more self-sufficient mentally to help to avoid illness, both mental and physical in the future. This should start by assuming that everyone is anxious from birth and all behaviour stems from this. To preserve their future health, they should be protected from shocks and long-term anxiety.

All this anxiety puts a strain on your immune system. If your nutrition is poor and your genes get switched on or off, depending how they are programmed a chronic disease will occur. How can we tell if someone is anxious? Read on...

5

HOW WE EXPRESS ANXIETY

Observation of a patient's behaviour, speech, expression, and dress allows the doctor to assess their anxiety levels. In conventional medicine, very little notice is taken of these things, as the doctor concentrates more on the physical symptoms, and their computer, but in homeopathic practice observations are made to a very detailed level, because this determines the choice of remedy.

We may notice the patient's gait on walking into the room, their speech patterns like loquaciousness, movements of the hands and feet, gestures, picking at the skin around a nail, facial expression and never sitting still. Fiddling with the hair and constantly pulling it can be severe enough to cause bald patches. Posture gives people away. If they are slumped, they give off messages of distress and depression and lack of energy. Tics and twitching of the mouth and eyes and eyebrows are usually associated with anxiety. The patient will be unaware that they are doing it. Nose-picking, lip-licking, closing the eyes, sucking the thumb in children, fiddling with jewellery and clothes, constantly moving hair out of the face, sweating, being too hot or too cold, needing to go to the toilet frequently, scratching. Even an itchy skin rash will be worse from anxiety. Nail-biting, thumb-sucking, and cramps and spasms all indicate lack of relaxation, even if they occur whilst asleep.

Patients with depression may have downcast eyes, very little movement, often wearing black clothes, and with gloomy thoughts and slower speech, as if the effort of life is too much.

The way someone dresses also gives insight into the way they feel. They may be scruffy and unkempt, or the opposite: meticulously neat and tidy, a perfectionist, not a hair out of place, and wearing smart, clean clothes. They may dress for comfort, or for fashion. Ladies may wear a lot of make-up, or none. Their clothes may be colourful, or all black. In this country, black is associated with death, so to wear all black must mean something to the wearer. Women may hide behind it and say black makes them look slimmer, which means that they are anxious about their appearance.

Dr James Tyler Kent, an American, asked homeopathic doctors from all over the world to send him symptoms and details of cured cases. He then compiled a repertory, which he used to write his book entitled *Repertory of the Homeopathic Materia Medica*, which was an amalgamation of all the information he'd gathered, and was first published in 1912. He divided the book into chapters according to parts of the body, and started with the mind, which he considered the most important. The mind section contains virtually every mental or character symptom that any patient could ever complain of or be observed doing. It contains lists of symptoms and aggravations and ameliorations. It is important to know what relieves symptoms and what aggravates them, because these details are very individual and may mean success or failure in prescribing the right remedy.

Each symptom has a list of remedies that have been known to cure that particular problem. These lists are called rubrics. Once a remedy has been decided upon, it can be checked in *Materia Medica*, which is a book containing the poisoning symptoms of every substance used for making medicines. Now the information in repertories is computerised. This is how homeopaths have always known that premenstrual syndrome symptoms which can be depression, anger and anxiety, are not a disease entity in their own right, but an aggravation of something that is already just underneath the surface, but suppressed by the body at other times of the month. The added hormone load at the end on the cycle causes the symptoms to arise. Whenever I've asked patients about this they always agree that this is how it is for them.

There are many words that patients use to express anxiety, but if the doctor has not learnt about homeopathy it is very unlikely they would pick this up, especially in GP, because even if the symptoms of anxiety were obvious there would be very little that could be done about it. There is no incentive to diagnose anxiety if there is no medication to prescribe as tranquillisers are highly addictive and rarely offered. Access to psychologists takes a long time, and the treatment they offer is lengthy with no guarantee of success.

It is rare that the patient sits down and complains that they feel very anxious. Mostly they complain of physical symptoms because they are used to dealing with a medical system, the NHS, which emphasises physical problems. The doctor, if they are interested, has to try to work out if anxiety is part of the presenting problem.

A patient took a list of symptoms to the doctor. She took a list because she was anxious that she would forget something that would turn out to be important for the doctor. The doctor was also anxious on being given a list, as he had not been taught to see a pattern of disease in it. Patients who bring lists cause worry for the doctor, and therefore are often referred to as 'heartsink patients'. The doctor's heart sinks when they see the patient coming through the door because they don't know how to cope with them, so really it is the doctor's problem, and not the patient's. I've been in another surgery and seen a poster on the window in the waiting room saying the doctor can only cope with one symptom at a time, so do not bring a list. I think this is a common experience for patients.

The doctor told the patient that he did not know what was wrong but he would send her for a blood test. If she had not heard anything in a week all was okay. As she did not hear she knew the test was all right, but as she still had the symptoms, she made another appointment a week later. The second doctor also could not interpret the list and said he would send her for another blood test in case anything had changed in the last two weeks. As she did not hear again after another week she showed me the list and asked me if I knew what was wrong. I told her that they were all symptoms of anxiety. She said she thought so, but why could the doctors she saw not tell her that? I prescribed some homeopathic arsenic alb. and her anxiety has been under much better control. She can now identify the symptoms of anxiety in herself and has some medication which helps.

Because of my homeopathic training, I had learnt that bringing a list of symptoms to a doctor can indicate anxiety, which is then easier to explore once you understand the pattern of presentation.

Everything that anyone says gives them away. The way that they say it also gives them away. Consequently, there is quite a long list of expressions we use, without realising that we are showing our anxieties. The anxieties may be very subtle like wanting to be liked, wanting to be one of the crowd, fitting in, wanting to be better than other people, or more knowledgeable, or boastful, exaggerating and feeling uncomfortable. Shouting indicates anger. People usually shout or swear when they have difficulty expressing themselves. This is an anxiety. They may resort to violence if provoked out of their comfort zone.

Anxiety can also express itself by shyness, timidity, avoiding crowds, avoiding strangers, stammering, difficulty in expressing yourself, rarely going out, not joining in, avoiding social interaction because it is too difficult for you, and you therefore may end up feeling

155

very lonely. It is easy to see how anxiety is behind all of this. People with autism always have the same patterns of behaviour, which reflects their way of coping with extreme levels of anxiety.

Once you assume that everyone, even babies, has some degree of anxiety, it ought to be a lot easier to have it diagnosed. With very little help to offer doctors are in a difficult position and they feel a duty to exclude physical illness first, hence all the blood tests and scans. If things are missed people complain or sue.

It is a problem to know with each individual patient whether the level of anxiety will increase, stay the same or be more manageable. It is helpful to discuss this with the patient because making a diagnosis gives patients insight. If they know that their doctor can't help much, they may go looking for help elsewhere and anxiety is the commonest problem seen in a homeopathic private practice along with respiratory and skin problems. Men rarely seem to complain of anxiety symptoms, and as they are not exempt from anxiety, they either bury it, or feel it is beneath their dignity to discuss it. It is therefore usually women who mention their symptoms.

If anxiety escalates panic attacks or mania can be the result. Mania is the result of your anxieties causing you to behave in a manic fashion which is an escalation of your normal behaviour. Your way of coping with anxiety is by talking and walking fast, spending money or other behaviours which have a calming effect on you. If panic attacks escalate then the patient may tip over into paranoia and delusions, i.e., severe mental illness. If the result of panic attacks is mania after a while this may tip over into depression when the patient is worn out and despairing.

As doctors it is very important to listen to the patient carefully, observe them carefully and work out their anxiety levels. Otherwise it is a missed opportunity. Even saying to the patient 'you seem very anxious' can be a help because it gives patients insight into what the doctor is focusing on. The patient then has an opportunity to talk.

What Might The Patient Say?

For acute, severe anxiety the patient might say they had such a nasty shock that their heart missed beats, they couldn't breathe and felt as if they were gripped in a vice. Some people faint from shock, as on receiving bad news.

They feel fear and panic as the adrenaline circulates round the body. They may need to go to the toilet urgently to open their bowels. They are left numb, speechless and sweating and then go very cold. They may faint and if their worst fears are realised, they can go into a fugue state which is when rational thinking stops and people wander round in a daze. Their brain seems to shut down for a while. If their worst fears are confirmed, their acute shock turns into post-traumatic stress disorder, which is a severe mental breakdown in functioning accompanied by night terrors and poor sleep with anxious dreams and a reliving of the awful event. As a consequence of this long-term the patient is more likely to get a physical illness as a direct effect on their immune system.

Unfortunately, post-traumatic stress disorder is very difficult to treat conventionally and is common in returning soldiers who have been in a war zone. It can be treated with homeopathy.

Anticipatory Anxiety

This can mean you're an early riser, which usually is due to fear of facing the day and what it might bring. Waking too early is very often misdiagnosed as a symptom of depression. There may be inability to eat breakfast because the stomach feels as if it is too tight to let food in, which is also part of anorexia nervosa. Anticipatory anxiety can also include worrying about everyday things, such as missing the bus, being late for an appointment, going up or, more often, down steps, bowel urging with loose stools, having to speak in public, and having to deal with a problem that feels too difficult to cope with, like a sick child at home to look after, or money worries. Children can experience anticipatory anxiety in the form of excitement before an event.

This anxiety can be bad enough to trigger an asthma attack or an exacerbation of any disease. The anxiety associated with day to day anticipation is very wearying and nearly always ends in some physical symptoms like irritable bowel syndrome. It is no use prescribing conventional medication for the symptoms of colic and looseness, because one medication will only treat one symptom. As homeopathy treats the whole person it is much more successful.

A man of 60 had been thoroughly investigated for his problem of burping, or eructation, having had an endoscopy and scans of the abdomen and brain. His specialist had not been able to find the cause nor any medication that would help. It transpired, although the consultant never asked, that he had fear of death as his brother had just dropped dead from a heart attack. Natrum mur. cured him within days.

Chronic Anxiety

Nearly everyone has anxiety to some degree, and it can be a day-to-day occurrence. It can be mild or develop into unremitting, more troublesome levels, still on a day-to-day basis, but can escalate into panic attacks. At this point it will become difficult to cope with, and affect people's lives. People express this as tension, nervousness, anxiousness, fearfulness, poor concentration, restlessness, insomnia, changes of appetite, feeling spaced out, and absent-minded, forgetful, inattentive, say they never have a chance to sit still and spend all day rushing around, become impulsive which may lead to a shopping spree and problems with money. Low-level anxiety may arouse jealousy and suspiciousness, or the opposite where people are known as comedians, which means that they desire appreciation to allay anxieties in the form of laughter or applause. Otherwise a person can develop an abnormal sense of control in their lives which means they are conscientious about trifles in their surroundings and must know where everything is and, in the extreme, become hoarders and never throw anything away as they worry that they may need the objects in the future.

With chronic anxiety people have difficulty making their mind up and will dither about decision-making, because change can make people fearful and anxious. Change includes moving house, going away to university, and having to cope with the important things in life like births, marriages and deaths. A newborn baby is anxious until its mother reassures it, and its mother may be anxious about how to handle it. This is the situation that can tip mothers into post-natal mental health problems.

People in pain are often scared of the implications of the pain – having a fear of chronic disease or death, and angry or worrisome thoughts such as, *why can't the doctors find out what is wrong and put it right?* Pain makes people tense up, which in turn makes pain worse. This took the pain-relief clinics a long time to discover, as they used to always look for a physical cause. It is the basis of fibromyalgia syndrome and polymyalgia rheumatica.

161

They seem to be similar conditions, but fibromyalgia is in younger people with severe anxiety and tension in the muscles, and polymyalgia rheumatica is in older people who have not got the resilience in their bodies of younger people and consequently develop a more severe version. If the muscles go into spasm from tension it is extremely painful and the patient cannot move. The treatment for PMR, never given for FM, is steroid tablets that are anti-inflammatory, which help, but can have serious side effects. Both disorders cause multiple tender areas which move around, so that some days the pain is worse in one spot and some days in another.

Phobic Anxiety States

A phobia is a persistent and excessive fear of an object or situation that is not always necessarily dangerous. The fear makes people avoid situations where the phobia occurs. Phobias are disabling as they interfere with normal activities.

Phobias are due to anticipatory fear of an event or experience that would make somebody anxious. If they are not anticipating being in a situation where the feared object will be found, like snakes or spiders, heights, or the sight of blood, they are not so anxious. A social phobia is when a person is anxious around other people, often because of a fear of judgement by them. An example is agoraphobia, which includes being afraid of going out or meeting others, and fear and avoidance of crowded situations that make the person increasingly anxious. Social phobias are becoming more common, and can make people lonely and lacking in confidence. They can all be treated with homeopathy.

Significant events in people's lives can be overwhelming and sudden which cause shock, or repeated, small and cumulative. If significant events are not rationalised by the person anxiety is the outcome and the phobic anxiety state is a protective mechanism. If the patient manages to come to terms with these events, they will get over the anxiety.

People feel threatened by things that make them feel anxious, and if something is anxiety-provoking it will be avoided or a pattern of behaviour will be learned to overcome the way in which the anxiety shows itself.

Expressions like stage fright, being crippled with anxiety and mute from anxiety are used to explain physical effects from anxiety. A patient went on holiday to France. She was driving and was all right for the first week, but the next day, whilst driving, she lost the use of one arm. She was taken to hospital and scanned in case she had had a stroke. Her brain was fine. In fact she was suffering from fear, and this had caused the paralysis. The driving was too much for her to cope with and her body gave her a paralysed arm so that she could no longer drive. Once she got back to England, she was fine. Fear also makes people stammer and break out in a sweat. Homesickness is anxiety of separation.

Even fish suffer from anxiety. Fear passes from fish to fish in a swarm, and they all leap out of the water. Animals can stampede from fear as can human crowds. Animals can die of shock, like sheep that have been worried by a dog. In this situation the word worried has two meanings – one mental and the other physical.

Fear, fright and anxiety can provoke or exacerbate many diseases, like bleeding in haemophilia, fits in epilepsy, skin rashes, tinnitus, morning sickness in pregnancy, menstrual disorders, vertigo, or irritable bowel syndrome. In fact, the more you tense up and become anxious, the worse any symptom will become.

Anger

Anger is a learned pattern of behaviour, and some people resort to it more often and to a higher level than others. The lowest level is being irritable about the small things in life, to the other extreme of being beside oneself, bursting with anger, a tendency to destroy things, and being bullying, abusive, violent and murderous. Rage makes people feel strong, the opposite of anxiety, as does being a bully.

People become angry when they are anxious about something that is outside their control. A good example is whilst driving in traffic. Some people are more easily prone to anger than others. Once people learn that anger can make them feel less anxious and in control, it may escalate. The NHS treats this situation with anger-management courses. There are many homeopathic remedies for people with different levels of anger.

Other words which indicate anger are indignation, sarcasm, arguing, and shouting.

Anxiety and Personality Change

Chronic recurrent anxiety can change people. We use words like anguish, brooding, full of cares, cautious, dwells on the past, inappropriate mood, which is usually when people laugh out of context and with a changed facial expression like looking haggard. It can make people restless, unable to sit down and rest, or concentrate. It can change people into someone who won't go on holiday or travel because it takes them outside their comfort zone; or make friends, and become too timid, and have difficulty making decisions.

A lady told me that during the Second World War her husband was in the navy. He spent a lot of time on battleships in convoys in the Mediterranean, the North Atlantic and the Arctic. He was due to rejoin HMS *Prince of Wales* when it was docked in Scapa Flow. As he was going up the gangway a man standing nearby beckoned him over. He was told that he was not going on this voyage but was being sent to London on a secret mission. He was asked to sign the official secrets act, and was unable to tell anyone what he was doing, including his wife. His wife thought he was on the Prince of Wales, which then left Scapa Flow and sailed all the way round to Singapore, where the Japanese bombarded it and it was sunk with all hands. As his name was still on the list from when the ship sailed his wife received a letter saying that there were no survivors. He was unable to tell his wife where he was and that he was safe. She grieved for him, and tried to work out how she would manage. Six months later he was able to tell her what he was doing and he wrote to her from New York. She had a terrible shock. It turned her into an anxious person unable to make her own mind up, or to make friends because she became very shy, and had difficulty coping for most of her life. She ended up with dementia.

People who need activity or become busy, because this seems as if they are using time well, are often exerting themselves because physical activity ameliorates anxiety. They may become impulsive or industrious and find that doing something makes them feel better. They become overactive, restless and sleepless and desire physical exercise. This may include sexual activity.

Memories are brain states that were imprinted in times past that you have to resurrect. If the memories are pleasant then no anxieties are associated with them. If, however, the memories are painful, they are associated with anxiety, occasionally, as in PTSD with severe symptoms.

Fear is a sense of danger or foreboding. The strongest fear is fear of death, for yourself and then family, which is why religion is so helpful to some people, especially when older.

The next commonest fear is fear of serious illness. This makes a visit to the doctor very anxiety-provoking. Cervical smears make people very anxious because of the implications of an abnormal result. I used to take the opportunity to examine patients and once people knew that things seemed normal a lot of anxiety went.

Other illness and situations that cause fear are cancers, strokes, heart attacks, AIDS, going blind, nervous breakdown, paralysis, pain, pregnancy, health in general, hospital appointments, impotence, infection/contagion, lung disease, surgery, pain, doctors, that you will not recover, respiratory disease, losing self-control, suffering, vertigo, and unexplained symptoms.

Depression

For some people, the anxiety they experience alters the way they think in that it turns them into a depressed state. The anxiety will still be there, but is added to by a state of anguish or despair or remorse, or a change of mood either completely or remitting, which means that you never know what mood the person will be in. The symptoms of depression can last from a few seconds at a time to long spells. They may be morose, lacking in self-confidence, weeping easily, causelessly or involuntarily, or the weeping provoked by things like music. Their mind becomes dulled, their pride takes a fall and they may feel victimised, undervalued and unfortunate. They may become complaining or talk to themselves. If the thoughts are compelling or persistent the person develops OCD as a coping mechanism.

When you lose control of your thoughts you may think only of death, despair and suicide.

Other symptoms of depression are thoughts like *why me?*, swearing, superstitions, suicidal thoughts, speech which is either loquacious or very slow, being secretive, sadness, guilt, which means reproaching yourself, brooding, complaining, pessimism, being gloomy, fretful, ill-humoured or sullen, moping, indifference, moaning, bad mood, mental exertion is impossible, menses aggravate, menopause aggravates, memory weak, loneliness, feeling low spirited, and kleptomania. There is also SAD, seasonal affective disorder, a form of winter depression.

Symptoms of depression may be part of the inability to adapt to change for a lot of people. This is one of the most important things in the lives of humans. How you adapt to change is one of the predictors of health.

Your view of others may also contribute to a feeling of depression, one of which may be contemptuousness, which means the person doesn't suffer fools gladly and is subconsciously saying, 'you stupid person, you', to get the upper hand. There may be strong feelings of cynicism, the patient may be dictatorial, haughty and insolent. He may resort to laughing contemptuously, mocking sarcasm, rudeness, and sardonic smiling. His view of himself may be one of eccentricity, extravagance, or reproaching himself. It is all an attitude of mind. Cognitive behavioural therapy tries to get the patient to see themself in this way and consequently to hopefully change patterns of thought.

Grief

Emotions and post-shock from grief or a severe event are:

1. Shock and numbness, and thoughts like, *I can't believe he has gone.*

2. Sadness and depression, usually for yourself. *How could he leave me?*

3. Tiredness and exhaustion from all the emotions, worry (*how will I cope on my own?*), and sleeplessness.

4. Anger, towards him for leaving you, towards the doctors who could not cure him, and to God for letting it happen. *Why me?*

5. Acceptance; depending on your nature, acceptance can be quickly resolved, can last years, or for a lifetime.

These emotional levels can be speedy or lifelong in their resolution.

The opposite emotions of tenderness, tranquillity, caring, compassion, empathy, a warm heart, friendliness, contentment, happiness, being fulfilled, optimistic that things will go right, joyful, satisfaction, contentment and things are good.

The definition of well-being, according to the WHO's mental health department, is a state of complete mental, physical, and social well-being. It is not just the absence of disease.

It would appear that anxiety levels are highest in the young and middle-aged, and the least anxious people are between 65 and 90. It involves being happy with yourself, feeling appreciated, and not living in the past. You no longer feel such a strong desire to achieve something, and have become wiser and more experienced. You probably have learnt to count your blessings, and have managed to adapt to change, and things that you found difficult to cope with. You have achieved a measure of tranquillity.

These feelings are also a reflection of your economic, social, environmental, and marital status in life, because these all have an effect on your anxiety levels. As you get older you no longer need to be tense, competitive, selfish, shifty, dishonest, distrusting, boorish, pedantic, unsentimental, arrogant or envious.

Compensation

If we lead a life full of anxieties, we need to find ways of compensating in order to lead a better-quality life. This depends to a greater part on how we are brought up. If we are in a tranquil environment which is calm and peaceful, we are much more likely to be calm ourselves. However, this also depends on how our genes endow us with the ability to cope. For each person nature and nurture will play a part, but in different amounts in each individual. It all depends on how our brains are wired up and how the circuits develop as we learn and grow up, our nutrition, and how our immune system matures.

If things are not going well, the person needs to find a way to compensate for the feelings that are difficult to cope with. This, in its extreme version, leads to addictions. For less difficult, but persistent anxieties, habits and behaviour need to change to try to adapt. This situation includes anorexia and bulimia. Addictions are the answer for many people. Addictions bring in another layer of problems to deal with as a result of the damage they cause to our health.

The consequences of all this produces people who are always early (anticipatory anxiety), or late, for appointments, become extravagant, do a lot of exercise, become fanatics, terrorists, fight, commit arson, steal, become fastidious in the extreme, or resort to childish behaviour, indifference, insolence, intolerance of others, which may be racialism, lying, libertinism, malicious behaviour, desire to make a noise... pop groups become easily offended, obstinate, untidy (hoarders), overactive, religious, zeal, superstitious, suspicious and talking too much.

A lot of these traits cause people to be different from others when they are excessive, as in people who are hoarders. Each hoarder will have a different background from other hoarders – in essence, they are all trying and failing to live a normal life, but have gone beyond their coping level and overcompensated because this is making their anxiety levels go down below their coping level.

This is a very important point for us all, as every disease and the happiness of your life depend on your coping skills.

6

THE INABILITY TO COPE SYNDROME:
Addictions

We saw in the last chapter that everyone has their own coping level and it is different in each person. Whether you go beyond your level depends on the circumstances of your life. It is not related to IQ, because exceptionally clever people are not necessarily good copers. It depends more on common sense, the ability to rationalise, and the ability to relax and not get anxious or worried, or stressed.

It is a common situation in general practice to be faced with a patient who says that they can't cope any longer, and is at the end of their tether. These situations forced me to think about coping skills and what it means to people.

If you are unable to voice your problem, or are not understood when you do so, how are you to cope? Friends and relatives may help with talking, but what if you cannot bring yourself to talk about the problem? Professional help is difficult to find and rarely available via your GP, so people resort to websites and charities.

What if you're a child, or someone whose personality (maybe shyness) does not allow you to express your problem, or if you feel ashamed about what is upsetting you, like bullying, for instance? What do you do then?

The major component of this syndrome is anxiety.

Trying to find a way of coping with your anxiety leads to addictions because people feel that whatever they are addicted to helps them to relax. The anxiety under these circumstances is usually described as stress. Stress stretches a person beyond their mind's ability to deal with the problem, that is, to cope. Everyone's coping skills are different, and it depends on our genes and life skills how we cope, but the major component is anxiety.

Babies

Learning to cope starts in the uterus. In previous times pregnant women were treated as delicate beings and allowed to do very little and told to avoid anxiety. Now they often work until the birth, and expect to have a calm and peaceful baby. Foetuses pick up maternal anxieties via hormones in the cord blood.

The baby next has to cope with its birth. If it has been anxious and restless, it may rotate and the cord can end up entwined round the neck. Semi-strangulation must be very anxiety-provoking during the birth, and so the heartbeat either reduces or speeds up, which is known as foetal distress. So an emergency caesarean section is performed, and the baby then misses out on picking up its biome from the vagina. A baby only picks up skin flora from a caesarean birth.

If the baby is not breastfed there is no opportunity to get its immune-system material from its mother. It then has a poor biome and low resistance, and so may easily develop problems like lactose intolerance, the first symptoms of which can be otitis media, or recurrent ear infections. The baby is then taken to the GP who prescribes antibiotics, which destroy the biome further, which makes the baby prone to more infections – and the cycle is repeated. This is very common in young children and also may be expressed in tonsillitis. Anything that is recurrent in babies and young children should be looked at in this way. It would be wise to tell the parents to avoid giving the baby lactose until it is better.

Case History: Baby with a Cough

Coughs are relatively easy to treat with homeopathy and in general practice the diagnosis is usually straightforward: colds or asthma. The diagnosis in this case was never made by GPs or paediatricians. I met the baby's granny at a funeral, and she asked me if I would see her daughter and grandson, as he was now 18 months old, and the doctors had been unable to cure his cough.

The next day the daughter told me that the cough had been present from birth. He was under the care of paediatricians and GPs, seeing a different one each time he consulted. He had been hospitalised three times for pneumonia and bronchitis. He had had X-rays and scans of his lungs and tests for cystic fibrosis, etc., but nothing had shown up. No one had diagnosed the problem by listening to him coughing, even when he was on the ward.

I asked her to describe the cough. She said that the minute he was born and drew breath he started coughing. She had not had a proper night's sleep since, as she was up so many times to him. He coughed so strongly that he could not get his breath, and then was sick at the end of the bout. That was a perfect description of a cough that needed the remedy drosera.

But there was a lot more. His mother was a busy lawyer and had a stressful job. At 34 weeks she had started labour pains and gone to the hospital. They gave her an injection of steroids and the labour settled down. However, the pains started again at 36 weeks and this time, despite two steroid injections, she continued in labour. She was then told that the baby was going to be premature and needed protection from infection, so they gave her an injection of the DPT vaccine, diphtheria, tetanus, and whooping cough. Ten hours later the baby was born coughing.

I don't know if the GPs and paediatricians had ever seen a case of whooping cough, but no diagnosis was made. The description of the cough told me what the problem was, as I had seen many cases. I gave him drosera and pertussin to take, and two days later she put a note through my door saying she had now had the first full night's sleep since he was born. Drosera was the commonest remedy used for whooping cough.

The night-time cough never returned, but as he was still coughing by day, his mum took him off dairy products and his cough went completely. She worked out that the antibiotics he had taken had wrecked his biome and caused the lactose problem.

I thought that the steroid injections had affected his immune system and consequently, when he had the DPT injection it caused the cough, because his immune system was unable to cope. A baby trying to get out of a stressful situation (his mother's stressful job) is already compromised. No one seemed to connect the events and no one recognised whooping cough, because, obviously, if you inject the mother with DPT you are providing protection not causing a problem. Why they thought a baby needed protection from tetanus, whooping cough and diphtheria is a mystery as there has been none in the UK for decades.

The interesting thing is that no GP or paediatrician had asked about his progress when he stopped attending because he was better.

The pathway of anxiety in the uterus, a stressful birth with foetal distress and possible emergency caesarean section, consequent poor development of the biome, lack of breastfeeding, leading to lack of development of the immune system, food allergies and intolerance, usually goes unnoticed by the doctor, so the baby develops failure to thrive and a vicious circle of illness. The way to stop it is to recognise it for what it is, stop all dairy products, add some live bacteria to the baby's diet, and treat any infections with homeopathy.

Children

I went on an introductory course in homeopathy and was given three bottles of homeopathic tablets to take home. One was arnica, the second was aconite, and the third was belladonna. I put them in my coat pocket and forgot about them over the weekend. On the Monday morning I was asked to visit a four-year-old boy who was very poorly with a high fever. He had been delirious during the night, and had a sore throat.

When I examined him, he had severe tonsillitis, glands enlarged in his neck, a high fever, a red flushed face, and he couldn't talk to me because it was too painful. His mother explained that he was having another attack of tonsillitis and had been having them every two months or so for a year. The doctor always prescribed penicillin, which took longer and longer to work, and he didn't get better for four or five days. During this time, he was unable to eat or drink, and had a high fever. She told me she was sick of it, i.e., her coping mechanism was failing, and it was about time the doctors came up with something to stop him having the attacks. Looking at the boy, I realised that he was showing exactly the same symptoms as those I had learnt about belladonna. I brought the bottle out of my pocket and asked his mum if she would like to try them. She read the information on the label, and realised the description of the indications for prescribing the remedy was identical to the illness that the little boy was showing.

She shrugged her shoulders and said she would try anything. I put a tablet in his mouth which he sucked. We decided to follow the instructions on the label, which said suck one tablet every 15 minutes until relief. I also gave her a prescription for penicillin, as I had no experience at that time of the homeopathic method of treatment, and no idea whether it would work or not. I told her to ring if there were any problems, and otherwise, I would see her on Thursday in the surgery.

On Thursday morning they turned up and I asked how he had been. His mum said she was astonished at how quickly the remedy had worked. She had done as asked and had given him one tablet every 15 minutes. After the third tablet, i.e., after half an hour, he sat up, said he felt a lot better and asked if he could have a drink. This was very unusual, as penicillin would never even have been absorbed into the body in half an hour. He was fine until about four o'clock in the afternoon, when he had a slight fever and his mum gave him another three tablets, after which he had something to eat. Most unusual for him. He slept well and had no hallucinations. The following morning, he had a slight temperature so another three tablets were given. He did not need any further dosage. His mum said she was very grateful for the rapid relief of his illness. She had put the prescription for penicillin onto the fire as she had not needed it. Not only did this episode of tonsillitis get better very quickly, but he never had another one again. This episode was so unlike anything that I'd seen before due to the speed of recovery, that I decided to try using homeopathic remedies in the practice for wider problems. I was very impressed, and often have been since, with the speed and depth of response.

Vaccines

At two months of age the first vaccines are given. At present there is no way of assessing which babies may develop side effects to them. Nobody considers that a history of foetal distress is important once the baby is born but it may have a lasting effect, like PTSD, especially when its immune system has to cope with vaccines. A two-month-old baby's immune system may not be developed enough to cope, and even at this point, the baby may already have eczema. All skin conditions are treated with ointments applied to the skin in conventional medicine, but if the eczema were seen as a reflection of an internal problem, as it is in homeopathy, doctors would consequently prescribe differently.

If a child feels unwell they become anxious, but will not always be able to express themself. Parents and doctors should all be aware of this.

Teenagers

A 15-year-old boy born in England, of Asian parents, had the severest eczema that the professor of paediatric dermatology had ever seen. He never had any relief from it and felt it was so unsightly that he wore clothes accordingly to cover it. His mother and father had had an arranged marriage, and his mother travelled to England alone at a young age where she knew no one and spoke no English. She was already pregnant when she arrived, and was very fearful and anxious. During the course of the pregnancy she had anorexia nervosa as a result of severe culture shock.

Within hours of him being born he started to develop eczema, and he was never free of it after that. He had antibiotics when it was infected, which was often. He could barely stop scratching and he was covered in scars where he had scratched. The skin was weeping and bleeding a little. He had been admitted to hospital a number of times for inpatient treatment, which mainly involved antibiotics and steroids usually by mouth and frequently on the skin.

Every time he went to outpatients, he had his blood tested for food allergies, and every time there were a lot of them and they were different. His mother was at the end of her tether and couldn't cope. His father was trying to support them and he was having difficulty coping, and the patient couldn't cope with his condition and his schoolmates' reactions to it, and so he developed a way of shutting himself off from his disease by spending his time alone in his room. The dermatologist couldn't cope either as the cyclosporine she had been prescribing for the last six months had not helped and had caused his creatinine to be raised as a result of damage to his kidneys.

The dermatologist wanted to change his prescription to methotrexate, but when the family read the potential side effects they declined and brought him to see me. The dermatologist was further perturbed by this, but had no other suggestions to offer.

It took me quite a long time to sort out what was really wrong with the patient, but it seemed to go back as far as his mother's pregnancy and her emotional problems. The eczema didn't respond to the first few remedies that I prescribed, although the remedy mixed of streptococcus and staphylococcus nosode (equivalent to a vaccine) helped infections. He took some prebiotics and probiotics to improve his biome, and his skin responded a little. It was not until him I gave him the remedy vernix 200C, three tablets sucked, one day a week, that he made progress.

After that things slowly improved. His consultant sent me a copy of a letter she'd sent to his GP, which said that against her advice I'd recommended he stop the cyclosporine, which I hadn't, and that his mother didn't understand the risks of taking or not taking the medication. His father in fact was very worried about his raised creatinine from the cyclosporine. She predicted that he would get a flare-up by stopping the treatment (as you usually do when you stop medication that is suppressing an illness). In fact, his father reduced it slowly whilst taking the homeopathic medication and there was no problem. The cyclosporin therefore could not have been helping a great deal. She predicted that there would be a severe exacerbation of his eczema and that it would not be a course of action that she would recommend.

The next letter to his GP said that she was very pleased to know that his eczema was well controlled just on homeopathic medicine. He was not using any other systemic treatment or topical steroids.

It seemed odd that she did not want to discuss with me what I had done for him as it was so effective, but I'm sure she was pleased to be relieved of the burden of having to make difficult decisions when conventional medication either caused problems or didn't actually work.

Mental Health Problems in Children

There has been a huge increase in mental health problems in children. The threat of looming exams is a problem, as is bullying and lack of self-confidence. Perceived stress causes release of adrenaline, which leads to exhaustion. Teenagers often get glandular fever at this age or at university, followed by post-viral fatigue syndrome. Doctors should realise that these are symptoms of being unable to cope, which existed before the glandular fever and so reduced the immune system so that illness was inevitable. Glandular fever is the body's way of saying stop. It can take a long time to recover from GF, and students can need a year off.

I met a man in the supermarket who stopped me and said he vividly remembered consulting me on the morning of 14th September 1989, when he was at school, and had a nasty sore throat. I had said I thought he had GF and asked him to go for a blood test. I also gave him some tablets of ferrum phos. 30C from the drawer in which I kept a supply of homeopathic medicines, and asked him to return the next day. When he did, I was able to tell him that he did have GF. I asked him how he was. 'I am better', he said. It made such an impression on him that

188

three tablets could make him better overnight, that he still remembered the exact date. I always found GF easy to treat with homeopathy and most people got better in 18 hours.

Teenagers now suffer from a variety of mental health problems like anorexia and eating disorders, and even young children can be poor and picky eaters, eating only a narrow variety of foods.

Anorexia is a troubled relationship with food. It can occur at any age. A lady of 92 was so fed up with her husband who bullied her, that she decided to live on whisky and chocolate, which she asked the carer to buy for her. She ate very little else and it took her two years to die. Her GP had no idea what was going on.

Anorexia is a serious mental illness which revolves around feelings of a lack of confidence and self-worth, which can be eroded by bullying, and causes severe anxiety. The feeling is that the person can't eat food as they haven't done enough to deserve it. Losing weight is synonymous with disappearing. It is the ultimate nervous breakdown and is exacerbated by an unhappy childhood and social pressure. It has a significant mortality rate. The brain needs to be rewired so that the sufferer can learn to

189

love themselves, and food, again. It can be helped by homeopathy, although the problem with this sort of illness is that people are sucked in to the system and go along the conventional route because no one ever suggests that homeopathy might help.

One point six million Britons are affected by eating disorders and feel that life is out of control and that they are not a tough or resistant person or they are not good enough.

Adults

When adults have severe anxiety and feel unable to cope they resort to finding their own ways of coping. This may include substances to which they become addicted, like cigarettes and alcohol. If you ask people why they smoke it is usually to help with anxiety. There are huge numbers of patterns of behaviour that people become addicted to often unknowingly, that will have knock-on effects on their health. Life is definitely a game of consequences when it comes to coping with the results of alcohol and cigarette addiction. Everyone must know that alcohol and smoking causes health problems, but that doesn't seem to be something that concerns people, as it is a long-term consequence, and the short-term consequence is the relief of anxiety.

If your life is full of stress, how do you learn to cope? Some things that people turn to are positive, like friends, and hobbies – including music, singing, walking, amateur dramatics, dancing and baking, etc. These are methods of relieving stress which don't involve addictions in the usual sense of the word. Some people like travelling and holidays to relieve their stress. People comfort eat, which may cause weight gain, or go off their food and lose weight. Alcohol can cause problems in teenagers and students if there is a culture of drinking in their society. On the other hand a lot of people drink every day and feel that just a glass of wine in the evening helps to relax and that they deserve it. After many years of drinking every day liver problems can emerge.

People say the same about chocolate; just a bar in the evenings – I deserve it and it helps me to relax. People who smoke say that they smoke far more when they are stressed, and it helps them to relax and not be so restless.

Exercise can have the same effect for some people. For example, running increases the release of dopamine in the brain which gives a feel-good factor. All sports produce an adrenaline rush, which people can become addicted to. Some people may consequently take part in dangerous sports for the effect that it produces.

The reasons for self-harm are more complicated, but they involve manipulation of thoughts, and produce the desire to cut as a source of relief.

Gambling also is very addictive, the consequences of which can be poverty. Hoarding also reflects a mental health problem from anxiety.

People often use recreational drugs and controlled drugs which the doctor prescribes to try and relieve them of symptoms of anxiety. Patients used to tell me that they took two paracetamol tablets at night to help them sleep despite the fact that they were not in pain and the paracetamol had no tranquillising effect, just placebo.

There is a growing increase of gender dysmorphia, especially in children. In the homeopathic book this is described as a delusion, which means that it is a mental health problem.

Other addictions include sex, violence, hair-styling, make-up, fashion, social media, plastic surgery, and botox.

Addiction to applause, which affects comedians, involves repetitions of self-worth for the recipient. Addiction to yoga and meditation can occur. In fact, anything that takes over life is an addiction if used to relieve anxiety and boost self-esteem. All these behaviours are available to look at online. There are teenage fan clubs online which cater for their addictions to cosmetic surgery. Anything that has big business behind it is not going to be bothered by ruined lives if their profits are vast.

If you feel safe, you are not afraid. If you do not feel safe and you are afraid, you are very anxious. The main fears in life are of death, the consolations of which are religion and obsession with diet. Fear of the dark, including ghosts, and nowadays, vampires and zombies, the consolation for which is sleeping with the light on. Other fears are of violence, of assault and of bullying. If the consolation does not ameliorate the fear, the person fails to cope and physical or mental illness occurs.

People who have addictions all have had problems in their past which have wrecked their self-esteem and put them in a situation they cannot cope with. They turned to their addiction to boost their ego or to reward themselves.

A young man of 19 had been diagnosed with schizophrenia, which had been provoked by recreational drugs. He was also a heavy smoker and was taking major tranquillisers for his problem, which left him feeling calmer, but dazed. He was currently living in a halfway house having being admitted to a psychiatric unit some months before. He had a very poor diet, mostly carbohydrates of poor quality and sugar, and was very overweight. He was aware that the recreational drugs triggered his hallucinations. Fortunately, he was very co-operative and could see the sense in eating a better diet, although no one in the psychiatric department had been interested in this aspect of him. His overriding symptom was severe anxiety and he had been constantly bullied at school. Homeopathic medicines prescribed helped his mental state considerably and over the course of the next few years he managed to eat better, and consequently lost weight, he regained some self-esteem, which meant he dressed better and got a job with prospects. He had realised that his anxieties were the underlying cause of his problem and understood that his illness was a consequence.

People who have addictions usually have had problems in their past which have reduced their self-esteem and put them in a situation that they cannot cope with. They turn to their addictions to boost their ego and to reward themselves. When it does reward them, it is self-perpetuating and difficult to reverse, which is why vaping has been so successful in stopping people smoking cigarettes.

Body image is a considerable problem for some people, often teenagers. To have a sense of belonging they may dress alike, go shopping, spend money on cosmetics and plastic surgery to improve their body image, have tattoos, which are now common, but used to be the province of ex-service men and prisoners.

You can become addicted to computers, either playing games or using social media, cleaning, hoarding, cars and speed, animals, and eating; 'life is good, let's eat!', reflecting either happiness, or that things are bleak and that food is your friend and a comfort. Being shy or introverted and scared to be around people makes you avoid them and new experiences and you find you cannot cope without a drink. Fear of being late is common and anxiety-provoking.

Things which cause anger include noise from neighbours, building sites, motorbikes, loud parties and music, and loud gardening machines and tools. Becoming angry may cause hate and violence, and its consequences when people cannot cope. Swearing is a consequence of a strong emotional charge and is used as an intensifier by people who have poor command of language and as intimidating tactics. People can also be addicted to abusing others physically, emotionally or neglectfully.

It is possible that brain cells join up in fractions of seconds, which reflect moment-to-moment changes in consciousness. Research shows that intelligent rats have large neuronal assemblies and pleasure-seeking rats have smaller ones. Humans who choose alcohol, drugs, dangerous sports, music with a continuous beat, or sex, are more likely to have small neuronal assemblies.

Various kinds of mindlessness are associated with enhanced dopamine brain levels and may be permanent. The plasticity of the human brain allows change. If you learn a language or mathematics, or play a musical instrument and read music, your brain cells grow more branches and increase connectivity. Thoughts matter and thinking personalises your brain. If the creativity is already established, taking recreational drugs may not damage it so much, because the brain is already programmed.

Modern medicine has a problem of poor understanding of addictions, and addicts are rarely treated by doctors as there is no drug available, apart from Antabuse, which when taken makes alcoholics sick if they drink. It is usually treated by psychologists, charities and groups like Alcoholics Anonymous, who rarely seem to understand the underlying problems, or if they do are unable to treat them. It depends on the person affected whether they can manage to cope with the treatment plans.

People who have addictions all had problems in their past which have wrecked their self-esteem and put them in a situation that they cannot cope with and they turned to their addictions to boost their ego or to reward themselves.

Bullying

The potential for bullying is considerable now, especially with the rise of cyberbullying, and affects many children's lives. People check their phones repeatedly and even at night, which can cause sleep problems. There is name-calling, insults online, hate mail, a daily barrage of abuse, and an influential class hierarchy at school, meaning some pupils are left out, bullied, and isolated. The child or teenager usually keeps quiet about it, especially to their parents, and tries to make – and hold on to – friends. The children's parents may not be interested anyway, and if the school takes no action either, the problem escalates. Children want to fit in with things like clothes and hairstyles. Bullies often notice this and make negative comments *about* their efforts to fit in, and the child can be left out of normal activities, especially at weekends – with constant erosion of their self-esteem. The bullied person loses hope and encounters despair, with a slow chipping away of their self-worth.

Internet

The Internet is impersonal. The bully does not see their victim's response. The despair may lead to suicidal thoughts. It is very damaging. Research shows that bullying in pigs restricts their growth, so has a direct effect on their brains.

Whatever your addiction, it is available online.

Obsessive-compulsive disorder could be classed as an addiction because the sufferer is compelled to do some action, which relieves anxiety and is therefore addictive. When people with autism and/or a learning difficulty have this problem, they can be admitted to residential hospitals to try to sort their challenging behaviour, as they are unable to speak about it. They often are discharged on tranquillisers, as a chemical cosh is the only way that they can be managed in society.

Money

Pretty much everyone has money worries at sometime in their lives. Having a lot of money can be just as difficult to handle, as for a lottery winner, as having too little. People can become obsessive about money. For example, people who are misers have severe anxiety about the future. Savers may also have anxiety about the future plus about getting into debt. Anxiety about owing money and fear of retribution from money lenders provoke a lot of anxiety and a lot of illness. People become unable to work as a result of being unable to cope. If they then turn to alcohol or drugs the problem intensifies.

If you also lack vital social skills like punctuality, the ability to shake hands, make eye contact, function well in teams and groups, are very shy, anxious, autistic, or have a mild learning disability, the chances of you getting a job are remote.

All addictions give relief or pleasure in the short-term, but there are always consequences. Taking drugs to relieve anxiety may push you into schizophrenia, for example. Smoking is risky, as is alcohol. Anything that you cannot do without in life means that you can't adapt, and adapting is the essence of an illness-free life, because it means you are coping. All animals have to try and adapt to their circumstances including humans. It is the way we evolve. Modern life now is much more difficult to adapt to.

Anxiety seems to be considerably more prevalent now, especially in young people. Record numbers are seen for self-harm, eating disorders, depression, etc. In 2015 emergency admissions for psychiatric conditions soared to double the number from 2011. There has been a 12% increase in chronic eating disorders. This is only the worst sufferers: underneath is a huge number of children that have less difficult problems, e.g., those who have less difficult eating problems and less anxiety.

The idea of competitiveness, exams to pass and grades to get causes some children a great deal of worry and is beyond their capability to cope. The bullies among this group resort to bullying as a mechanism to get themselves self-esteem. Anger and manipulation, and control of others are the only ways they can cope. Bullying was almost non-existent 50 years ago, presumably because most of the children were better copers.

It is very important to people to feel one of the gang, and copy each other's behaviour, like clothing, hairstyles, tattoos, cigarettes and alcohol. A good example of this is bikers. They make friends who have a similar outlook on life, which gives them confidence. When retired, people should join clubs like the U3A, the University of the Third Age, and meet people who live locally and share similar likes.

Coping mechanisms have to be learnt from early childhood. You either adapt (cope), or do not. If you do not, you suffer from burn-out, which I prefer to call the 'inability to cope syndrome'.

We live in cities with a fast pace of life, overcrowded roads and neighbourhoods with noise and speed. Some people are particularly sensitive to noise, as well as to smells, light, tastes, etc., and some people have their senses reduced or absent as in the case of deafness. If your hearing is blunted, for example by working with noisy machinery or musical instruments, without using defenders it can lead to hearing loss. It may be also that your auditory nerve can be switched off by not actually wanting to hear, which is like switching your mind off to bad news.

There are too many people for this planet to support, so there is competition for education, jobs, partners, having it all, money, luxury, territory, which is why a lot of people want to emigrate, not only to get away from wars and dictators.

Competitive people may get angry that others cannot do things as well as they can. This puts pressure on people to work harder, do more hours and they feel stressed and anxious and exhausted.

You can also be addicted to your work. When you retire and it is taken away from you, you can feel bereaved.

Universities

There are up to five suicides a year at the top universities. Why do some students find life so difficult now?

Medicine was a tough, five-year course, and we started out with 90 students in my year, 25 of whom were women. When I taught students homeopathy at Birmingham University, there were 400 in each year and the 20 in my group had never met each other before. The medical school was not big enough for so many students, so they were placed in GP practices around the area as soon as they started. This meant that they had no early grounding in the basics. The students wanted to see patients, not get stuck in laboratories. In general practice patients were selected for them who, for example, had had a heart attack. The patient described the symptoms, and the students then studied the anatomy of the heart, the physiology of the heart, the histology of the heart, and so on. The next patient had kidney disease and the same method was taught, which meant that systems were never connected. They learn their anatomy not from dissection but from computers, in 2-D rather than 3-D. It also meant that GPs became teachers some days a week, and did not see patients.

We were taught anatomy by dissection, physiology, histology, bacteriology and pathology for two years before we were allowed onto the wards to see real patients. We therefore had a thorough grounding in the basics. We then did medicine, surgery, paediatrics, obstetrics and gynaecology, pharmacology, orthopaedics, ENT, ophthalmology, and all the other disciplines with the relevant exams along the way, before finals. During the final year we did (unpaid) locums for the current house officers who wanted a holiday. So by the time we qualified we were very experienced.

As a postgraduate, the first hospital I worked in had no A & E, but I did a one in two rota, and when on call took calls from GPs who wanted patients admitting urgently. I looked after two 35-bed wards, one male and one female, and was not allowed to refuse an admission. There were no specialist units, so I took everyone with every possible diagnosis, including MIs, strokes, asthma attacks, pneumonia, malignant hypertension, acute leukaemia, septicaemia, and everything else. My consultant, the registrar, the nursing sister and I did ward rounds every morning, including Saturdays, at 8.30 a.m. The consultant sat and read the paper whilst I had my breakfast, as the junior staff were all in residence. I may have had only a few hours' sleep but still had to get up for the ward round. At the end of the round I had a long list of blood tests, ECGs, X-rays, lumbar punctures, and so on, which needed to be done. I had to do them all myself as there were no technicians. There were not even any ward clerks to fill the forms in. By the time I got into general practice five years later I had done six months' medicine, six months' general surgery, six months' obstetrics, six months' paediatrics, one year in medicine in Nigeria during the Civil War, six months' gynaecology, six months' nephrology, and quite a lot of GP locums. So that by the time I went into general practice I could tackle the vast number of patients to be seen daily – up to 35 per surgery. My coping skills were well developed.

Now, all doctors work in specialised units, and there is no general medicine or surgery as such. There are over 45 different specialities and the same number in paediatrics. So, once the patient has been seen in A & E, they get transferred to the speciality they need. Consequences of this super-specialisation are that surgeons have been able to develop techniques that would never have been dreamt of years ago, to the benefit of the patient. I must say that the body of the elderly man that we dissected had an implant of ytterbium in his pituitary gland that had been inserted via his nose and had shrivelled his tumour. This technique has hardly changed in 50 years, other than it is now done by someone who specialises in it, and does no other surgery, rather than by a generalist brain surgeon. It is a sign that this tumour is now much more common than it used to be.

We were trained to cope and if you weren't sure about something, you asked the registrar in hospital, or your partner in GP. When I did paediatrics there was no registrar, only the consultant and two SHOs, so you had to be confident and reliable.

Now that MIs are dealt with in another town in our area and taken there by the paramedics, it is possible that you could enter general practice without ever having seen a patient with one. You may therefore have had training in resuscitation, but no practical experience. The patient comes out of hospital on medication, beta-blockers, statins, aspirin derivatives, etc. Your physical problem is dealt with skilfully if you are taken to the right place. If you are woman and your heart attack presents different symptoms, you are less likely to get this efficient treatment. No one, however, asks you what led up to your heart attack.

Young doctors now work shifts. They complained that working one in two, or one in three rotas were too tiring, and tiredness causes mistakes. My generation, however, was of the opinion that ignorance and lack of experience cause mistakes, rather than tiredness. When we joined the EU, we had to abide by its rules about doctors working hours, and consequently our hospital doctors started working shifts.

The most difficult thing in medicine is dealing with patients, taking histories, and making diagnoses. If doctors can't cope with the work they leave, seeing patients to others, and go into anaesthetics, laboratory work, haematology, bacteriology, pathology, genetics, research, etc., or leave medicine altogether and go into writing, journalism, TV, comedy, acting, join a drug company, or go into a business like running nursing and retirement homes. Shouldn't all doctors have to give a number of years after qualifying to the NHS?

Face to face with patients is very difficult and you need to learn to read patients and ask the right questions. A teacher comes to see you just before Christmas with bronchitis. She looks worn out and says she's had a very stressful and anxious term with two members of staff absent. She knows what caused her bronchitis but having it confirmed and talked about, rather than just being told it's a virus, is very helpful and only takes a few minutes. Because doctors are not coping so well, diagnoses of this sort are being missed frequently, which would be an opportunity to discuss causes rather than just prescribe antibiotics or tell patients that, 'it's just a virus'. Homeopathic treatment of coughs is very helpful and often produces a very quick result.

I was called to see a family of six children with coughs in the 1980s. I lined them all up to examine them and the nine-month-old baby was propped up in the corner of the settee. Whilst I was listening to their chests the baby started coughing and ended the spasm with a whoop. Mum said their coughs were all the same and there was whooping cough in the road. She knew there was no treatment and dreaded looking after six children with whooping cough because it would mean a lot of disturbed nights for weeks and she would not be able to cope. She was very interested when I offered homeopathic medicines. Some weeks later she brought them all down to the surgery to thank me for getting them better so quickly over a few days. Her neighbours had asked what her doctor had prescribed that had got them better, as their children's coughs had taken six weeks to improve. Studying homeopathy was a big help to me, as well as the patients, in coping with their problems

If coping mechanisms have to be learnt in life, it presupposes that the patient can learn. People who are severely anxious like autistic children may take a lot longer to learn than people who are confident.

Being unable to cope may be called a nervous breakdown. It comes when people are at the end of their tether. Anxiety releases adrenaline and acetylcholine increases when nerve signals overreact. Acetylcholine esterase is released to counteract this. It is a possibility that this system may be faulty in ME as this system controls muscular activity. The patient may say, 'I'm a prisoner of my fear', or 'I become paralysed from fear'.

Exhaustion is a common presentation in general practice, usually described as being tired all the time; or, in GP parlance, TATT. Serious physical illness must be ruled out, but once having done so it is generally caused by the inability to cope.

Fibromyalgia syndrome used to be called fibrositis.

Symptoms include:

- Multiple tender areas mostly along each side of the spine, arms and legs

- Increased sensitivity to pain

- Fatigue

- Muscle stiffness

- Sleep problems

- Mental problems like brain fog, poor memory and concentration

- Headaches, often from a tender area in the neck or forehead

- Irritable bowel syndrome

Conventional treatment is analgesic tablets with injection of the tender areas with local anaesthetic and steroids, antidepressants, sleeping tablets, muscle relaxants like diazepam, anti-epileptics, and antipsychotics.

It is easy to see how stress and muscle tension could cause this problem. Patients used to say that we all have a weak spot in our bodies and illness shows itself there.

It is treatable with homeopathy by paying attention to the underlying emotional problems.

Young men who are not coping (rarely women) develop risky or stupid behaviour like fighting, climbing up and jumping off mountains, aggression, seeking dangerous locations, dressing up as clowns and scaring people, and driving round with car windows open, shouting at people as they pass to give them a fright. Some of this behaviour may land them in trouble either with the police or with injuries if weapons are involved.

Essentially, most people are nice, decent, trying to make a way in life, and show a little kindness and respect. Discussion can be the solution to a lot of problems.

Peace and quiet is boring to the young. People look for recognition, applause and a pat on the back. Happy, well-adjusted pop stars are rare.

A lot of people have commitment phobia and cannot settle to what they see as a routine, well-ordered life. People want instant gratification, but those who do well in life can manage delayed gratification.

Doctors are now in business to make money and profit from people's anxieties, as in private practice. Specialists can charge £250 for a 30-minute appointment, which usually ends in the patient having investigations and a further, expensive appointment. This is one reason why general practice is not as popular as hospital medicine for doctors, as there is no private work in GP any longer. In GP, money is made from employing nurses to do follow-ups for diabetics and asthmatics, vaccinations, especially for flu, and medicals for people with a learning disability.

In business there is a rule about the inability to cope; called the Peter Principle, it states that people are promoted to do a job which is beyond their competence (ability to cope).

Violence

Children who are subject to violence, or witness it, develop different reactions when threatened. The normal reaction is fight or flight, which increases the heart rate, causes a clenching sensation in the stomach, dilated pupils, and a strong desire to open the bowels. This is the normal reaction to shock. The abnormal reaction is dissociation, which causes coldness of affect. The child is vulnerable and never feels that it is safe to depend on anyone. Unless you can bear your own vulnerability, you cannot accept it in anyone else. This can be addictive and acts like an antidepressant. The consequences can be sadism.

Food affects your brain from feedback from your biome via the vagus nerve. A poor diet means poor mental health.

Dopamine is usually released from the brain constantly, but when an event is better than expected the rate increases to give a feel-good experience. When the event is worse than expected the amount decreases.

Willpower

The 'I want it now' syndrome. Delayed gratification as a result of increased willpower curbs the emotions.

Nervous Energy

When you are nervous (anxious) your body produces enough energy for you to run away. If you do not have to run away the energy is not used, and the consequence is exhaustion.

Personality

Which is the more important in the formation of your personality? Genes or conditioning? The more positive your outlook, the longer your life. Optimism is very powerful, and the ratio between optimism and pessimism determines your health. 'Always look on the bright side of life.' A negative outlook on life affects everything. A negative outlook is mainly worry – *what if?*

The amygdala in the brain deals with threat and fear, and the autonomic nervous system deals with arousal levels. They can be measured in the electrical conductivity of the skin and the pulse rate.

The tendency to be optimistic or pessimistic is 50/50 genes and environment. Your genes are not fixed and switch on and off. The hippocampus in the brain is involved in anxiety/depression, stress, emotions and memory. Your memory is closely connected to your emotions. Many areas of the brain are involved and the experience of anxiety is different in everyone, which is why there are so many different remedies for anxiety in homeopathy.

The brain of a baby rat is modified by the care it gets from its mother. The better the care, the more glucocorticoid receptors it has, and the same applies in humans.

Your personality subtly changes and modifies throughout your life. People mellow with age. On the other hand, the brain cannot cope when there is low IQ, poor education, and a poor home environment.

The physical body cannot cope, i.e., the internal organs, if it constantly has to detox alcohol or chemicals, nicotine, etc. The lungs cannot cope with toxic inhalants, the liver and kidneys cannot cope with alcohol, and the bowel (biome) cannot cope with sugar and low fibre.

However, consumerism persuades us to eat and drink things that we should not, with an expectation of life that cannot be achieved. Big business does not care about our well-being.

Body Image Problems

There has been a 1,000% increase in incidence of gender dysmorphia in the last ten years. There is also a link between gender dysmorphia and autism. Autism is seven times more common in people who want to change sex. This may reflect a lack of ability to accept oneself. There is also a link to homosexuality, in that 60% to 80% of boys who asked for gender change are homosexual or bi-sexual.

The issues will not change with a sex change. The growing demand reflects damaged children. What do the follow-ups of these children say about the outcomes of gender reassignment? Too early to know? Do they get followed up for many years or just re-referred if problems arise?

Good mental health means being in control of your mind and emotions. Poor mental health means your emotions and mind are out of control. You are continually out of your comfort zone and lack confidence. Men may feel shameful and weak. This may happen to sports people after an injury, when they can't take part in their sport, i.e., are unable to cope. Sports people feel that ego is a sign of strength and inability to cope is failure of the ego, and causes depression.

Retirement may cause the same problems in that the person comes to the end of old certainties and has to rely on themselves, particularly if they live alone.

Dementia

In a study by GPs in Stafford, published in *The Journal of Family Practice* in 2013, it was shown that anxiety (plus depression) is a premorbid risk factor for dementia. Other risk factors were smoking and alcohol, and cardiovascular disease, all of which are symptoms of the inability to cope.

Big pharma has been notably unsuccessful in finding medication for dementia after 20 years of research. This is a consequence of looking at the body in terms of the function of one organ or part of the organ in its smallest detail, and not looking at the whole person. If the cause is the brain shutting down to stop anxiety, reflecting neural plasticity and wiring of the brain, then they are never going to be able to find any medication, unless they come up with non-addictive tranquillisers that people can take all their lives. Just like Soma in *Brave New World*.

7

INFLAMMATION, MICROBIOMES, NUTRITION, AND DIET:

Inflammation

Inflammation is the basic healing mechanism and the body's natural reaction to invaders or disease. It produces the four cardinal symptoms of rubor, which is redness, dolour, which is pain, tumour, which is swelling, and rigor, which is fever. Think of a boil. If the symptoms are part of the body's natural defence mechanism, why should you take anti-inflammatory medication, like ibuprofen, if the body is trying to heal itself? You are preventing the normal function of the body by doing so, and suppressing the natural reactions of the body. Most painkillers have some anti-inflammatory action, the first one put on the market was aspirin, but this is rarely used now as it has so many side effects.

If you have a chronic disease like arthritis, there is likely to be more long-term damage from taking anti-inflammatories, as these suppress inflammation so the problem does not heal. It just provides temporary help. The ideal way to treat inflammation would be by homeopathy, as this encourages the inflammation and consequently heals very rapidly.

As an example, we were taught about research done in the 1950s which showed the sequence of events seen on microscopy of coronary arteries when occlusion was developing leading up to a heart attack. Circulating bacteria want to reproduce, and to do so attach themselves to the wall of the artery. The body senses this and causes local inflammation to try to kill the bacteria. Inflammation causes swelling and consequent turbulent flow of blood over the surface of the swelling. This is also sensed by the body, which sends cholesterol to smooth over the swelling and produce laminar flow. But calcium is laid down in the cholesterol which builds up and eventually causes a blockage.

The main problem is circulating bacteria. The more sugar in the body, the more the bacteria grow. Bacteria are grown in laboratory conditions on sugar solutions. Professor John Yudkin in London in the 1970s said that anyone who wanted to avoid heart attacks should not eat sugar.

Consequently, cholesterol is only an indirect cause of heart attacks, and in fact is part of the healing mechanism.

Most gallstones are made of cholesterol and they are formed by the body in response to bacteria in the gall bladder. The cholesterol will engulf the bacteria and kill them.

Inflammation is initiated when the body sensors pick up invaders, or something which is in the wrong place at the wrong time, or when there is faulty nutrition which causes absence of vitamins and minerals or trace elements, or when there are other bodily reactions like allergies and intolerances, or the start of cancer changes in cells. Any abnormal metabolic pathway will cause inflammation. The body will try to put this right via the immune system and moving nutrients from one part of the body to another, but if the diet is poor, this will not be possible. The brain controls all this via the immune system, but the brain needs to be healthy, which includes thoughts and nutrition, to cope. The internal milieu is in delicate balance, and if not robust enough to cope, will cause symptoms of disease.

A diet rich in foods that help the inflammatory process will naturally help a lot of illnesses, like rheumatoid arthritis and osteoarthritis. Foods which help the inflammatory response are oils like olive and avocado, omega-3 oils found in fish and nuts, fruits, vegetables, garlic, herbs, spices like turmeric and cinnamon, soya, peppers, wholegrains, green leafy vegetables, dark chocolate and green tea.

Your Biomes

Once your food has been swallowed it is broken down by the acid in the stomach, it has bile added to it from the liver, then enzymes for digestion from the pancreas, and it ends up in your small intestine to be absorbed. Your small intestine is full of live bacteria, some of which are good for your health and some of which are unhealthy. If the healthy bacteria outweigh the unhealthy bacteria you will be well. If it is the other way around you will be ill.

If the unhealthy bacteria are more abundant, they damage the lining of the bowel and cause microscopic holes to appear in the gut wall. This is called leaky gut syndrome. If you've got leaks you can absorb bigger molecules than you would normally do. This puts an enormous strain on your immune system and it is overworked. The first problem you are likely to develop under these circumstances is allergies and intolerances. Hay fever, asthma and eczema are all aggravated and may be caused by an abnormal biome. Gluten and lactose intolerance or allergy problems are all improved by attention to restoring the natural biome.

Damage to a Biome

Unfortunately, the gut biome is damaged by quite a number of drugs. The main damage producers are antibiotics. They kill off the good bacteria in the gut as well as the pathological ones you are taking them for, like acne. The pathological ones left in the gut overgrow. Often the one that is left in the gut is candida, which is not a bacteria but a yeast. Overgrowth of candida in the gut causes thrush in the mouth in babies, vaginal thrush in ladies, and itching around the anus in men. If these conditions occur the whole gut should be treated and not just the local problem. This usually involves taking anti-fungal medication for a month from the GP. Live bacteria should be taken at the same time to restore the natural balance. Homeopathic remedies also restore the correct balance.

The next commonest medication group to damage the biome is proton pump inhibitors, PPIs, like esomeprazole, lansoprazole, omeprazole, pantoprasole and rabeprasole. The drug manufacturers make so many different compounds because when the patent runs out and any company can make the medicine, they can come up with another one so they still have the monopoly. The new one is marketed as being superior. These are given to people with stomach complaints like reflux, to reduce the amount of acid secreted. They also damage the biome, therefore should not be taken for long periods of time. However, this is the most widely prescribed group of drugs across the world and is commonly given to patients for their whole lives, because modern medicine cannot cope with the underlying problem in any other way.

The H2 blockers that also reduce stomach acid like cimetidine, famotidine, ranitidine and nizatidine also affect the biome, and should not be taken for long periods.

Another common damager of the biome is food additives. The main ones that cause problems are emulsifiers which improve the texture of food and lengthen its shelf life. Once they are in your gut, they alter the mucus coating that lines your gut and so damage the biome. They are

223

used to mix an oil with water, as in ice cream and mayonnaise. Some are natural, but some are synthetic, and the synthetic ones change the biome by covering the villi in the small intestine and stopping the bacteria from functioning. Other things that affect your biome are smoking, alcohol, vinegar, stress, and parasites including candida (thrush).

The condition of having the wrong bacteria in your gut is called dysbiosis. It was first discovered by Dr Edward Bach, the bacteriologist at the Royal London Homeopathic Hospital in 1926. He wrote a book about the bowel nosodes, which is still in print. A nosode is a remedy made from a pathological substance like a virus, bacterium, blood, etc., and acts like a vaccine. He took samples of patients' stools and made homeopathic remedies from the bacteria that he discovered there. The remedies were given to the patient to help them recover from their illnesses, and are still used in the same way. There is one called the poly bowel nosode that is prescribed for people who have had antibiotics to help repair damage to the biome.

Further work was done on this subject by doctors John and Elizabeth Paterson at the Glasgow Homeopathic

Hospital in 1960. They showed that abnormal gut bacteria reverted to normal after treatment with homeopathic remedies when the patient was better.

It is only recently when people with severe hospital acquired infection with clostridium difficile were treated with faecal transplants from healthy people because antibiotics had caused the problem in the first place, so couldn't be given again, that doctors have taken an interest in the biome. Modern researchers should read these early works and should also look at Dr Russell Malcolm's book *The Bowel Nosodes Reappraised* from 2002. It is full of information about the relationship between diseases and bowel flora and how they can be treated with homeopathy. There is a nosode for clostridium.

Ever since Koch and Pasteur saw micro-organisms under the microscope, we have been trying to rid our environment of them because some of them cause disease. Big businesses have produced strong household chemicals to keep hospitals and the home aseptic. However, disinfectants cannot tell the difference between bad and good bacteria and kill them all, to the detriment of our biomes. We breathe in the air around us which contains all

225

the natural bacteria that our guts need. Inhaled bacteria end up on the back of our throats and we swallow them down into our guts. This apparently is why a country walk makes you feel good, because you breathe in bacteria from sheep, cows and horses, and this improves your biome.

Doctors should tell every patient who has antibiotics and PPIs that they must heal their biomes. This involves sugar-free diets and lots of live bacteria, either from live yoghurt or capsules. They should also eat food with a lot of fibre which helps the bacteria to grow. Fermented foods like sauerkraut and miso are also good for restoring the biome.

If this does not work then parasite cleansers are available from the alternative market. Parasites are not only worms, but the wrong bacteria, and viruses and thrush.

Leaky Gut Syndrome

When the altered bacterial balance in the gut damages the lining, microscopic holes appear in the villi. Larger molecules than should normally be absorbed are absorbed. This puts a strain on the immune system as well as sending messages to the brain about toxins. This scenario is thought to be the explanation for such a large increase in allergies that patients are suffering, including asthma, eczema and rhinitis, hay fever, coeliac disease, and lactose and gluten intolerances.

My research in general practice showed that nearly everyone who had endometriosis had had antibiotics, often long courses for acne, recurrent tonsillitis, or cystitis. The gut and therefore the immune system was damaged, and this was apparent in the peritoneal cavity in these patients, because they did not reabsorb the endometrium spilled from the fallopian tubes during menstruation, which is what endometriosis is.

It also appears that dysbiosis may be responsible for obesity, as your biome affects how much energy your body takes from your food. Via the vagus nerve, hunger signals are made by the brain, and cause cravings according to your mood. This is a natural cycle, as the gut bacteria can convert foods to a range of chemicals and hormones, which affect our mood, appetite and general health. Therefore, if you suffer from depression you should alter your biome.

The Vagus Nerve

The direct brain-gut connection is via the vagus nerve. It is the 10th cranial nerve from the brain, and is the longest nerve in the body. It is a mixed nerve with motor and sensory fibres.

The nerve fibres going to and from the glands of the mucous membrane of the pharynx, larynx and the organs of the neck, mostly the thyroid plus the heart, lungs and abdomen, provide a feedback system and keep everything under control. The signals also regulate renal function and glucose control.

The vagus nerve can be stimulated by slow, rhythmic diaphragmatic breathing, humming and chanting, speaking, singing, washing the face with cold water, and meditation. It also helps to balance the biome.

Having a high vagal tone means that your body can relax faster after stress. It means better functioning of many body systems, decreasing blood sugar, which causes less risk of stroke and cardiovascular disease.

It also helps better production of digestive enzymes from the pancreas, and a better mood with less anxiety and more resilience.

A low vagal tone is associated with strokes, cardiovascular disease, depression, diabetes, chronic fatigue syndrome, cognitive impairment, inflammatory conditions and autoimmune diseases including rheumatoid arthritis, ulcerative colitis, endometriosis, thyroid disease, and lupus.

The sensory fibres pick up signals from the respiratory tract, pharynx and oesophagus, and the visceral fibres from the lungs, heart and the abdominal viscera.

So, there is a direct connection between the brain and the gut, and the better condition your biome is in, the higher the vagal tone. The gut starts at the mouth and ends at the anus. This means that doctors should consider all the symptoms – from the mouth to the anus – to have an emotional connection, for example, mouth ulcers, teeth grinding, throat clearing, eructation, reflux, and peptic ulcers. Before we knew about Helicobacter pylori, all peptic ulcers were considered stress-related. H. pylori cannot be the *cause* of peptic ulcers. What about the people who harbour HP but never get an ulcer? The consultants call this a pre-ulcer condition and treat it with antibiotics. You are told you will get an ulcer or even cancer if you don't treat it. They try to eliminate H. pylori, but in a few years it could recolonise the stomach, and will not produce symptoms. It should be considered part of the biome. Ironically, if you want to eliminate it, a course of antibiotics is prescribed, which kills off the abnormal biome in the stomach and wrecks the biome farther down in the small intestine. Consequences are rarely considered.

Other gastrointestinal problems associated with stress are irritable bowel syndrome, haemorrhoids, anal splits (fissures) and anal spasms.

Irritable Bowel Syndrome

If your abdominal pains, indigestion, reflux, flatulence, and distension have been investigated, and food intolerance or allergies ruled out, you will be offered antispasmodics like loperamide for the pain, and Gaviscon for reflux. You may also have diarrhoea or constipation, or alternating looseness and constipation. There is no treatment for wind and distension. The usual cause in this situation is anxiety and stress, and it is very unlikely that your GP will treat this aspect of your problem, as they have nothing to offer in the way of medication.

How should it be tackled? I did a small study in general practice which showed that homeopathy was an effective way of treating IBS.

IBS is usually treated with an antispasmodic, mebeverine, for colic, which is an old-fashioned medication derived from atropine that was extracted from atropa belladonna, which is toxic and used in the homeopathic medicine belladonna. Diarrhoea is treated with loperamide, also sold as Immodium, which is an opioid, similar to codeine, the side effects of which are abdominal cramps, constipation and abdominal bloating. Constipation is treated with laxatives. My patients with IBS all had single homeopathic remedies which covered all their individual symptoms, as everyone has different varieties of symptoms and different background causes.

One lady was so impressed with the results that she volunteered to come to the medical school when I was teaching homeopathy, to students to talk about her experiences with IBS. She told the students that the homeopathic treatment had given her life back as her symptoms had been so bad, despite taking the prescribed medication, that she had been afraid to go out of the house, and had to know where all the toilets were when she did.

The balance of different microbes in our gut reflects our individuality, our medical conditions, past history, and the food we eat. The best food to keep your biome healthy is high-fibre and multicoloured, which includes vegetables, herbs and spices, and brown bread, pasta and rice. Wholegrain products include the husk of the wheat that provides fibre and chromium, which the body needs to make insulin-resistance factor, which is missing from white rice, which may explain why so many Asian people are diabetic.

Eat only food you've prepared yourself.

Take probiotics in capsule form or yoghurt without sugar or make your own yoghurt. Add prebiotics which are oligosaccharides found in onions, garlic, wheat and beans, and inulin which is found in fibre. Avoid antibiotics and medication which suppress acid.

Eat plenty of fibre and multicoloured food, and inulin, which is found in leeks, onions, garlic, root vegetables and bananas. Eat nuts and seeds, green tea and dark chocolate, olive oil, unpasteurised and blue cheese. Eat live yoghurt and fermented foods like sauerkraut, pickles, kimchee, miso, and tempeh.

The Biome

1. Controls the formation and memory of 85% of the immune system and is the fundamental driver of the body's defences.

2. At night it consumes a kilo of yeasts and microbes that enter your body with food, and is the first line of defence for the immune system.

3. Makes B vitamins, vitamin K, and short-chain esters.

4. Is vital for your DNA replication and for controlling your homocysteine levels, a high level of which is a marker for heart disease and cancer.

5. Protects your liver and stops bad cholesterol formation.

6. Controls inflammation and even kills cancer cells.

7. Helps remove toxic compounds from the body.

Foods which affect the biome harmfully are sugar, cows' dairy, saturated (animal) fat, coffee, gluten, and chemical toxins like fluorine. These foods change the pH of the gut and favour the pathogenic (bad) over the commensal (good) bacteria.

When the balance is out of order the yeasts make holes in the lining of the gut wall and allow chemicals, toxins, allergens and yeasts to invade into the bloodstream.

People with chronic illness lose volume and diversity of the biome. Because of the inflammation caused by the chronic disease, the immune system is active elsewhere and the biome suffers.

Conditions linked to leaky gut syndrome are diarrhoea or constipation, fatigue, pains in muscles and joints, bloating after meals, burping, flatulence, mouth ulcers, thrush, cystitis, yellow toenails, Crohn's disease, IBS, lupus, diverticulitis, autoimmune disease, depression, eczema and allergies, so far.

It seems ironic that when you have recurrent cystitis caused by E-coli from your biome that the doctor gives you frequent courses of antibiotics, which alter your biome further.

Heal Your Gut

It should take about three months to heal your gut. This involves eliminating bad bacteria by eating plenty of garlic, cinnamon, oregano, curcurmin, herbs and spices, and all-natural compounds that kill yeasts. Pathogens are killed by cloves, slippery elm, and black walnut. Products containing these substances can be bought in health-food shops or online. To restrict the growth of bad bacteria and encourage good bacteria, take probiotic capsules containing acidophilus, lactobacilli and bifidobacteria. You must include L. rhamnosus to heal the holes. There is not enough in live yoghurts. You also need prebiotics, which are found in fibre in food.

To replenish the diversity of the good bacteria in your gut, eat sourdough bread, sauerkraut, Japanese foods, including seaweed, and apple cider vinegar. All oils, seeds and nuts will provide the right nutrients.

To increase the volume of the good bacteria, eat prebiotics like apples (*an apple a day keeps the doctor away!*), pears, onions and chicory, and take a probiotic, which is best bought in capsule form. Heat and damp kill bacteria, and a minimum of eight billion per day is required.

To heal a leaky gut eat glutamate, found in chicken soup, Methylsulfonylmethane (MSM), which helps joints and ligaments, essential fatty acids, found in omega oils, aloe vera, magnesium, vitamin E, and curcurmin. Exercise helps, as does inhaling the essential oils of lavender, thyme, cumin, and peppermint.

Vitamins and Minerals

- Are absorbed in the gut, but if there are none in food (for example, there is no selenium in the soil in the UK, so there is none in the plants that are grown here), you will not have much in your body. Selenium is an anticancer mineral.

- Nutrition helps mind and body.

- Supplements improve the IQ of schoolchildren, especially picky eaters.

- Phosphatidyl serine supplements help improve age-related memory loss.

- Nut supplements help ADHD and autism.

- Zinc supplements help anorexics.

- High-dose multi-nutrients, especially vitamins B3 and C, help schizophrenia.

- 5-HTP supplements help depression, anxiety and insomnia.

- As Patrick Holford states in his book *Optimum Nutrition for the Mind*, there is a 35% decrease in aggressive behaviour in prison inmates given vitamins, minerals, and essential oils.

Biomes in other Organs

Biomes are not only found in the gut, but in the breast, mouth, vagina, renal tract (bladder, kidneys and prostate), skin, and, possibly with further research, will be shown to be in the liver, ovaries, endometrium, spleen, testicles, brain, gallbladder, appendix, and pancreas, as well as all the glands. If the biome in the breast is out of balance because it is constantly affected by chemicals like parabens in deodorants, and the person's coping levels are exceeded by a sudden shock or continuous stress, then cancer will develop if the nutritional levels are poor.

If you have a poor biome in your mouth, which is altered with mouthwashes, toothpaste, a poor diet and poor condition of the teeth, this will also cause disease.

Sugars

Professor John Yudkin wrote his book *Pure, White and Deadly* in 1976, telling us that sugar causes a lot of illness. It has taken many decades for us to heed his warnings.

Biochemically, sugars are any compound whose name ends in 'ose'. This includes sucrose from cane sugar, glucose, fructose from fruit, maltose, dextrose, xylose, lactose (milk), and mannose.

High-fructose corn syrup, also known as glucose-fructose syrup, is cheap and a frequent ingredient in our food, particularly ice cream. It causes fatty liver disease and accelerates the growth of cancer cells. Fatty liver, which is also common in alcoholics, is a fundamental cause of insulin resistance and diabetes. It accelerates the growth of cancer cells.

Insulin's functions are complex, but its primary role is to promote the absorption of glucose into body cells. A high-sugar diet causes release of more insulin and at some point, your cells will resist and be unable to function, which is what type 2 diabetes is. People who are overweight are considerably more at risk of becoming diabetic, and if you are diabetic and overweight you are more at risk of complications.

How much sugar is safe? This is the same question as asking how many cigarettes are safe. Sugar is toxic. A healthy diet avoids sugar and refined carbohydrates like white flour, pasta and rice. The huge incidence of diabetes in China, India and the USA is probably as a result of eating white rice and white bread. Because there is no chromium in white food and insulin needs chromium to function, it therefore cannot function properly. Doctors seem to be unaware of this.

Sugar should be classed as addictive, and if you replace sugar with fat, you lessen the cravings for carbohydrates. The yeasts in your biome depend entirely on sugar intake for their growth.

When nutritionists were not part of mainstream medicine, they wrote books about the biome and thrush and health long before it became better known to doctors, who mostly poured scorn on the idea. Hospitals don't employ nutritionists; they've always employed dieticians which are not the same. I once suggested to a local gastroenterologist about a patient he was treating that she should have her biome treated, and he said he didn't believe in it. So, I continued my own way, advising everyone who had antibiotics to avoid sugar and pay attention to their guts – especially when on antibiotics. I was the only partner in the practice who advised patients in this way.

When I came to write about endometriosis and polycystic ovary syndrome, which are related to diabetes, I always advised patients to pay attention to their biomes. They were very grateful to get this advice and could see the logic, but found a low-sugar diet very hard, as sugar is so addictive.

Polycystic ovary syndrome, which I call the 'tough ovary syndrome', is also to do with a poorly functioning immune system as a result of a poor biome, and causes local pelvic problems, but just on the ovary. The capsule of the ovary becomes thickened and doesn't allow ovulation, so multiple cysts form as an ovum matures but is not able to get out of the ovary. This causes infertility and should be treated in the same way with attention to the biome and avoidance of sugar.

Sugar promotes inflammation in cells, which may be one reason why people go down with respiratory illness at Christmas.

Vaccinations

We no longer suffer from cholera, polio, smallpox, measles, whooping cough, and more, but have acquired a huge increase in chronic diseases instead. Cross-contamination in families should occur naturally, and when children used to suffer from infectious diseases their biomes were healthier. This was immunity acquired from contact with viruses, which had been with humans since we evolved on the planet. Now we are vaccinated against all these diseases with altered viruses. How does our immune system deal with abnormal viruses that we are not evolved to deal with? Someone should do some research on the biome of newborn babies and how it changes after vaccination.

The less you go out, the less new bacteria you pick up and consequently your biome depletes. This may well be an important reason why people who are confined to home and rarely go out develop chronic diseases.

If you feel better in the countryside than in a city, it means your biome population is happier and more diverse.

It is important to keep your biome intact. So, avoid anything that will damage it, which includes mouthwashes, chemical toothpastes, and antibacterial soaps; to bring up your child in the best of health, try and avoid caesarean sections, which now account for 25% of all UK births. The long-term effect on the biome will be huge. Biomes are transmitted down the generations by infections, not genes. Babies born naturally are covered with vaginal and anal bacteria from the mother. This gives it a complex dose of maternal bacteria, that is, the start of a healthy biome.

Hygiene

It is always interesting to me to see programmes on the television about cleanliness in the kitchen, when swabs would be taken and the homeowner informed of what dreadful bacteria were lurking there. It struck me that the people were not ill as a result of this. People's bodies had adapted to having these potentially pathogenic bacteria about and they produced a healthy biome which coped. Soil in the garden contains healthy bacteria, which is why gardening is good for us. Keeping a house clean using chemicals alters the biome and introduces toxic chemicals into the environment.

If you have a healthy biome you will absorb more nutrients than if it is unhealthy. The consequences of not absorbing nutrients is disease.

Nutrition

Vitamins, minerals and trace elements are the essential building blocks of life and good health. Most are found in fruit and vegetables. Proteins, carbohydrates and fats should contain as many of these as possible, and provide nutrients for repair and healing of all the organs of the body.

Genes contain instructions for making proteins in the body. Proteins make enzymes which do the work of turning one chemical into another. Enzymes in turn are activated by nutrients. If you have a defective enzyme you may need more specific nutrients. If you are lacking in some of these nutrients, your body is not going to function as well as it could.

To produce optimal functioning of different organs, a wide variety of nutrients is required. For the brain, vitamins A, C, D, and E, which are antioxidants (antioxidants deal with the waste products in cells), and the vitamin-B group. Fats, including omega-3 and 6, and phospholipids plus amino acids, glucose, and oxygen from the atmosphere are all essential. To make neurons and neurotransmitters function you also need choline, serotonin, adrenaline, noradrenaline, dopamine and GABA (the tranquillity neurotransmitter). The amyloid plaques which build up in the brain of people suffering from dementia are abnormal proteins which can also be found in the plaques of arterial deposits in people with coronary artery disease. This is not to say that the amyloid is the cause of the disease. It is more probably a consequence of inflammation.

The measurement of the level of homocysteine in the blood is an indication of your risk of heart disease and stroke. Unfortunately, this is not available on the NHS.

The lower the level the better your nutritional status and the better your body is at manufacturing necessary chemicals. These bodily chemicals like acetyl choline, serotonin, dopamine and GABA are neurotransmitters which keep your whole body functioning, using the principle of psycho-neuro-hormono-immunology.

The brain also needs essential fats, mostly derived from fish, phospholipids, amino acids, and vitamins and minerals like zinc and magnesium. You should include oily fish and sunflower seeds in your diet. If we overfish and experience global warming, the consequence will be that we are unable to eat the raw materials for the functioning of our brains.

Good fats are essential. If you have been on a low-fat diet you will be missing some essential health-giving nutrients. You should eat less dairy fats and more nuts and seeds, and oily fish. Eat salads with olive oil on them. Eating eggs is important, because although they do contain cholesterol, eating them doesn't raise your blood cholesterol level. Cholesterol is essential for good health because of its anti-inflammatory properties. Your brain contains large amounts of it, and it is used to make the sex hormones oestrogen, progesterone, and testosterone.

People with a learning disability, like Down's syndrome, and people with chronic disease need to keep their brain in top function. It is a good idea to supplement with lecithin granules, as this helps to make amino acids in the brain.

Protein is vital since all neurotransmitters are made from it. The body needs 23 amino acids to build everything from neurotransmitters to a neuron. You eat only the eight essential amino acids because the body can make the rest from these. Fish, chicken, eggs, and tofu (from soya) contain the most protein of the best quality.

Mental Health

All the vitamins and minerals and trace elements are key nutrients for intelligence and mental health. Vitamin B1 deficiency shows itself as poor concentration and attention. B3 deficiency causes depression and psychosis, B5 poor memory and stress, B6 irritability, poor memory, depression, and stress. All of these vitamins can be found in wholegrains and vegetables. Folic acid deficiency can cause anxiety, depression, and psychosis. Folic acid is found in green leafy vegetables, and doctors should advise all pregnant women to take it, as well as women trying for a baby. It can prevent spina bifida, as it is needed to build a healthy brain and nervous system.

Vitamin C deficiency causes depression and psychosis, and is found in vegetables and fresh fruit.

Magnesium helps muscles relax, painful periods, angina, and general relaxation. It also helps premenstrual syndrome, which is irritability, insomnia, and depression. It is found in green vegetables, nuts, and seeds.

Manganese deficiency causes dizziness and convulsions and is found in nuts, seeds, tropical fruit and tea.

Zinc deficiency causes confusion, blank mind, depression, loss of appetite, lack of motivation and concentration, and poor development of spermatozoa. It is shown by having white spots on the fingernails. It is found in nuts, seeds and fish.

The B group of vitamins and vitamin C are water-soluble, and pass through the body and out in the urine, so we need a regular intake during the day.

Calcium and magnesium help to relax nerve and muscle cells. They also help you to sleep.

The gut produces two-thirds of serotonin, the happy neurotransmitter. Good nutrition is not just about what you eat, but is also about what you can digest and absorb, and how well your genes prime your metabolic processes.

1. One of the main factors in absorption of vitamins and minerals is stomach acid. As you get older you produce less. The acid is necessary to start the digestive processes in that it breaks down the food you eat. Stomach acid production depends on zinc and you need to produce a hormone in the stomach called intrinsic factor which allows absorption of vitamin B12 from your food. Lack of intrinsic factor causes folic acid deficiency and pernicious anaemia, and vitamin B12 needs to be given by injection every three months.

2. Lycopene, an antioxidant found in tomatoes, reduces cholesterol and blood pressure. It helps with the flexibility of arteries and the sensitivity of blood vessels to oxygen, which is a vasodilator. It decreases LDL proteins, which is bad cholesterol, and reduces triglycerides and blood pressure. Harvard Medical School showed that eating ten helpings of tomatoes a week, preferably cooked, could reduce prostate cancer risk by 40%. If you already have

the cancer, it could still reduce the symptoms by 40% as well.

3. Selenium is deficient in British diets as there is none in the soil. There is very little in Europe either. It's one of the most important anticancer minerals and deficiency has been linked directly with stomach and breast cancers. It is known to increase cellular oxygen and glutathione peroxidase activity. The best source is Brazil nuts. It is also found in garlic, tuna and oily fish, onions, sunflower seeds, tomatoes, wheatgerm, eggs, and chicken breast.

4. Zinc helps antioxidants like vitamin A and C to do their jobs. It accelerates healing time. It is found in seeds, wheatgerm, shellfish and garlic, and is depleted by alcohol. Dairy products block its absorption.

5. Potassium, found in lentils, broad beans and peas, wholegrains, nuts, bananas, fresh fish, green vegetables, brown rice, carrots, apples, pears and oranges, is found in every cell in the body, and enables the mitochondria to produce their energy. Without potassium, cells will adopt a different method of functioning and may become cancer cells.

6. Vitamin D acts as a regulatory hormone. There are a large number of vitamin D receptors in the body and it can kill cancer cells. It can adjust almost everything in the cell, from its genetic messaging, to its cytoskeleton. It can even switch genes on and off. Everyone, and particularly cancer patients, should spend 40 minutes a day in the sunshine and/or take a supplement. It is made by the action of sunlight on the cholesterol layers below your skin (do statins damage this layer?). A small amount is found in oily fish and even less in dairy. It is thought to offer protection from 15 different cancers, including breast, prostate, colon and pancreatic. It also helps to break cholesterol down and acts as an anti-inflammatory. (Would it be better to take vitamin D supplements rather than statins?) We make most of it from sunshine. Fish oil is an anti-inflammatory and helps keep triglyceride levels normal. It helps the body deal with inflammation and protects against coronary artery disease, and is also found in pumpkin seeds, shellfish and garlic. The French say that if your breath does not smell of garlic, you are not healthy! This is probably the ingredient in the Mediterranean diet which keeps the locals healthier than we are in Britain. Vitamin D blood levels predict survival

from cancer. The lower they are, the less likely you are to survive.

7. Coenzyme Q10 helps to produce energy in cells. It is mostly found in active tissue like muscle, brain, heart and kidneys. Levels decline as we age but supplementation can restore levels to those we had when we younger. The amount in the body can be considerably reduced in people who take statins to reduce cholesterol levels, and bisphosphonates for osteoporosis.

Diets

A diet is manipulation of eating habits in order to achieve a change in health. The well-known ones are for losing weight, using different methods of calorie intake like fasting, low fat, low carbohydrate, and overall reduction in the amount eaten.

Less well known is the acid-free diet. This is designed to make your blood more alkaline. Blood pH is normally about 7.4, and if it is higher than that is alkaline, and if it is lower than that it is acid. The food you eat creates an acid environment normally, and the most acidic thing you can eat is sugar.

Osteoporosis

The conventional medical view is that all elderly women, but not men, have osteoporosis. If they do, why does everybody not suffer symptoms from it? Why do people who have osteoporosis, which is a decrease in bone density and therefore bone mass, not lose weight? It is a known side effect of people on steroid medication, for example for asthma and polymyalgia rheumatica. That must include men.

The NHS recommends a diet high in calcium from dairy products, with vitamin D supplements, hormone replacement therapy, and bisphosphonate tablets and injections, which are prescribed as etidronate, alendronic acid, ibandronic acid, risedronate sodium, and strontium ranelate. Risk factors for osteoporosis include smoking, previous history of anorexia nervosa, low weight, previous history of steroids, high alcohol intake, no physical activity, family history, early menopause, and hyperparathyroidism, which is overactivity of the parathyroid glands.

I once asked a rep who was selling new bisphosphonate tablets by how much he would expect the bone density to improve after a year's treatment. He didn't know the answer, but said he would get back to me, which he never did. I therefore assumed that this aspect of treatment had never been studied. The American gynaecologist Dr John Lee prescribed natural progesterone cream made from yams for his patients, and said that their bone density increased by 4% per annum.

Professor Jane Plant says in her book *Osteoporosis* that bones are like rocks. If you put them in an acid medium they dissolve. The main acid producing foods are dairy and sugar. Dairy products are cows' milk, cheese, yoghurt, ice cream, etc. They also contain cow oestrogen, and this foreign hormone promotes breast and prostate cancer. It is possible to manage without dairy as there is plenty of calcium in green vegetables, nuts and fruit. Dairy products should be substituted with soya, almond or oat products, which are plant-based and easily available. The natural progesterone in your body, even after the menopause, plus the plant oestrogen in soya products, will turn it into human oestrogen, which stimulates bone renewal. In Southeast Asia women rarely get osteoporosis because they eat very little dairy products and a lot of soya.

If you increase your salt intake you excrete more calcium. Excessive parathyroid, thyroid and adrenal glands hormones (adrenaline from stress) are a risk for osteoporosis as is an early menopause or spells of amenorrhoea from over-exercising, as in athletes.

Drugs that cause osteoporosis include thyroxine, heparin, warfarin, cyclosporine, cortisone, anti-epilepsy medication, gonadotrophin-releasing hormone used for infertility and endometriosis, aluminium in antacids, and aromatase inhibitors which are given to postmenopausal women with breast cancer.

An acid-free diet is mainly plant-based with low carbohydrates and proteins, and is a diet that would suit many other diseases including diabetes. Despite what people think, fruit and vegetables are not acid-producing, despite some of them tasting sour. A typical Western diet causes a chronic state of acidosis.

Osteoarthritis is a metabolic disease, not a disease of wear and tear or old age, which means an acid-free diet will help it. Abnormal metabolism in the joints causes

254

hydroxyapatite to be laid down in the cartilage, which causes minute holes to appear. These small holes get bigger and eventually the cartilage is shredded and the raw surfaces of the bone rub against one another, which is what osteoarthritis is. It also responds to an acid-free diet, but the damage may be done.

Rheumatoid arthritis is inflammation of the synovial membranes lining the joints. It is generally considered to be autoimmune, caused by your own immune system, and is now common in children and young adults. It also is helped by diet, with anti-inflammatory herbs and spices like turmeric and ginger, garlic, onions, asparagus, fresh pineapple and oily fish. Food intolerance is common in people with rheumatoid arthritis – particularly dairy and gluten. There is a possibility of viruses or bacteria in the synovial membrane. It responds well to homeopathic medicine.

Skin diseases like acne, dermatitis, eczema, psoriasis and psoriatic arthropathy all improve on an acid-free diet.

All diseases of the gut will improve if attention is paid to the health of the biome. In fact, an unhealthy biome is a precursor for colon cancer. Crohn's disease and ulcerative colitis are commonly associated with lactose sensitivity, though an acid-free diet would be helpful. Avoiding milk avoids any bacteria carried in the milk. Milk is high in histamine and contains carrageenan, which is used to stabilise milk proteins, and this can cause gut problems.

An acid-free diet has been shown to help multiple sclerosis, breast, prostate and gastrointestinal cancers, depression, anxiety, deep vein thromboses, clots, autism, ADHD, food allergies, sensitivities and intolerances.

8

EXTERNAL FACTORS:
The Toxic Environment; VOCs

We live in a world full of pitfalls for humans. Modern science has invented many things that have an impact on health, from coal mining to computing. Environmental pollution is a common cause of illness. It is possible to avoid a lot of pollution, but first the pollutants need to be identified.

One of my friends died from lung cancer. He was asked by the consultant about smoking. He had never smoked, and neither had any members of his family. He was told that the histology of his cancer showed a variety of lung cancer not caused by smoking, and that now only three out of five lung cancers are caused by smoking. Two out of five are not. What are people inhaling now that is causing lung cancers?

Why is the incidence of asthma increasing so rapidly? In fact, all respiratory disease is increasing, despite fewer people smoking.

Everything humans do affects the environment – including building houses, roads, quarrying, and manufacturing. Manufacturers are not going to stop their lucrative businesses because there may be possible health problems, which are not even scientifically proven. Annual sales are enormous, with Nestlé (Nescafé, KitKat, Nespresso, Purina) leading the way, with £72 billion sales, and Proctor and Gamble (Ariel, Gillette, Oral-B, Fairy, Tampax) second, with £52.6 billion.

Outdoor Pollution

Outdoor pollution is mainly diesel fumes which cause 23,500 deaths per year from nitrous-oxide pollution, pollen and fungal spores, which cause asthma and COPD – chronic obstructive pulmonary disease, which used to be called emphysema. If you use the London Underground the air pollution is so high, that there is a risk of lung disease. Tube travellers can inhale more than 12 million tiny, toxic particles a minute. This nanodust is mainly iron oxides from train movement. It is also thought to be a risk for dementia.

Diesel fumes have been reclassified as a grade one carcinogen, which means that they are a definite cause of cancer. It is estimated that 650 people a year die from cancer caused by exposure to diesel fumes at work.

If your neighbour has a wood-burning stove they could be harming your health. It behaves like diesel fuel and releases billions of the tiny, toxic particles into the air, which drift into nearby houses. They account for 31% of toxic particles in the air. Other environmental problems are caused by cable lines, mobile-phone masts and Wi-Fi, which is electro-magnetic radiation.

Big business dumps toxic waste that it cannot get rid of, as Monsanto did in South Wales.

Arsenic is found in the groundwater in Argentina, Chile, Mexico, California, Mongolia, China, Bangladesh, Vietnam, Thailand, Taiwan, Hungary, and Romania. Rice grown in these countries needs to be cooked in a large amount of water to remove the arsenic. A trial of treatment with homeopathic arsenic was done in West Bengal in 2005, as the usual methods of removing the arsenic from the groundwater were not very effective. Arsenicum album 200C was given to people who promptly excreted high levels of arsenic and their blood levels dropped. Standard chelation therapy was not as effective. Arsenic could be in baby rice, rice crispies, rice milk, and rice biscuits bought in the UK. In homeopathic practice you look for a remedy that could cause the illness that the patient has. Arsenicum album, white arsenic, is a common remedy for anxiety.

Animals

Cows eat grass and turn it into methane and carbon dioxide, which are expelled into the atmosphere and are greenhouse gases. Their meat is used to feed dogs and cats, as well as humans. The market for pet food in the USA is huge, as there are 163 million dogs and cats as pets.

Global Warming

World ecosystems, like coral reefs, are disappearing. Half the world's fish depends on coral reefs. Global warming is established and causing reduction in Arctic ice and the spreading of deserts. The sea temperature is increasing. Population lies at the base of many of these problems. Not enough food is being produced to support the global population, and consequently people are migrating. The air is polluted, which aggravates global warming. Flooding and drought are causing problems. Dust storms are a consequence and these cause asthma. Particles from storms are small enough to go through the alveoli into the bloodstream. They are mostly silica and calcium sulphate, calcium carbonate and quartz, which are tiny, sharp crystals, mica, pollen, and bacteria.

The oil industry in the Middle East needs water, so dams are built, which dry up rivers and lakes. This effect is worldwide, with rivers and lakes disappearing in a lot of countries. The war in the Middle East aggravated the dust and added toxic particles to it.

Desertification needs to be tackled with native plants to prevent further erosion. There should be satellite data available for water management to control soil moisture, which can inform farmers about the need for irrigation with a global, early warning system for dust storms. The deposit from these storms can be beneficial as it can provide valuable nutrients for plants.

Asthma

Episodic wheeze occurs in 30% of children worldwide, even in island societies where there are fewer cars. Persistent wheeze occurs in 10%; 75% of all asthmatic children are atopic, i.e., allergic, and 50% of asthmatic adults are. The rest are sensitive or irritated by things they inhale.

Indoor Pollution

Indoor pollution is mainly hidden and not considered as a cause of disease. There are too many chemicals in our environment, offered to us to clean our houses and ourselves. They are designed to smell nice, but the smell is the problem.

VOCs
(Volatile Organic Chemicals)

Volatile means they give off a smell, usually called 'perfume', 'parfum' or 'fragrance' on the list of ingredients. Parfum is a combination of chemicals, often more than a hundred, designed to smell 'morning fresh', or whatever the manufacturers think customers will respond to. The commonest products that contain these VOCs are detergents, softeners, products that go in dryers, aftershaves, perfumes, room fresheners, toilet cleaners, household cleaners, furniture fresheners, most sprays, cosmetics, soaps, shower gels, bath bubbles, shampoos, lipsticks, toothpastes, deodorants, etc.

Many VOCs are carcinogenic, e.g., acetaldehyde. Not all are found on the ingredients lists. As well as asthma and eczema, they can cause fits and neurological diseases.

The Best Smell is No Smell

When you wash your clothes, linen and towels in detergent, it is designed to smell of the chemicals in the formula. The smell is manufactured to stay in the clothes, and every time you wear them, your body warmth makes the clothes smell. The smell is the VOC, and you take it around with you everywhere and sleep in the sheets at night.

You constantly live in a toxic, chemical fug. You don't notice it yourself as your nose stops sending messages to your brain after a short while. You never get rid of the smell. These chemicals irritate the skin, so if you have eczema or any skin rash, don't use them. Either do without, or use Ecoballs in your washing machine, which also saves a lot of money.

The chemicals are absorbed through the skin and lungs and end up in the liver, where the body tries to detox them. Having to continuously detox these chemicals puts a strain on the liver. If you add in alcohol the liver is in trouble.

When you breathe these toxic chemicals in they stay on the back of your throat, so they are swallowed. They end up in your biome and alter the balance of good and bad bacteria. They are excreted through the bowel and also the kidneys. As far as I know, none of this has been scientifically investigated as a cause of disease, so your consultant is not going to tell you to avoid them. However, I have cured a lot of people who have asthma by advising avoidance of these products.

Avoidance

Unfortunately, supermarkets have an agreement with detergent manufacturers to put their products in a prominent position on the shelves, so that they are at eye level and you cannot miss them. You never find alternatives to detergents displayed as a result. There is no need to use detergents in your machine. It is possible to use Ecoballs, which get the dirt out by ion exchange and not chemically. They are sold online. They are considerably cheaper to use than detergents, which is why the washing-product manufacturers are not keen on them. If there is a stubborn stain use the stain remover supplied with the Ecoball. You will save a lot of money and not put toxic chemicals into your own environment and anyone nearby's environment when standing next to them. The residual water will not put chemicals into the water system from your washing machine.

It is possible to buy most personal cosmetics as free-from toxic chemicals. The VOCs in shampoos, bathroom products, hair dyes, and deodorants can all be avoided. It means reading the ingredients lists and knowing the chemicals to avoid when shopping. If you have an asthmatic or someone with respiratory disease in the house they will be helped considerably.

If parfum can cause asthmatics so much ill health, could they not also cause lung cancer? Has anyone tested them on humans?

The chemicals in shampoos can cause hair loss. The patients to whom I have suggested slowly stopping shampoos and washing with water instead, have all had less itchy scalps, less hair loss, and thicker, more manageable hair. There seem to be a lot of young girls who have problems with poor hair growth. If you put toxic chemicals on your scalp, including hair dyes, it can damage your hair roots so that your hair falls out.

All these chemicals we use also end up in the environment. It is known that flame retardants used widely in the 1970s in furniture and mattress manufacture suppress the immune system and can cause cancer, mainly thyroid in adults and cognitive deficits in children, and are behind bacterial and parasite infections in animals, and reduce their fertility. There has been a 74% increase in thyroid cancer in the last ten years.

VOCs are also found in tobacco smoke, paint, and paint remover, varnishes and wax, pesticides, air fresheners, glue, cosmetics and shampoo, printers and copiers, wood-burning stoves, fuel oil, and gasoline, furniture, and carpets (when new), detergents, and car exhausts.

Do the doctors who do IVF, or specialise in male and female fertility, look at the toxin loads of their patients? Male sperm counts have dropped by 50%. Over a thousand stranded dolphins, whales and porpoises were tested and found to have very high toxin levels. If that is so in these animals, what must it be like in humans? Who tests humans? Why do the vets know more about it than doctors and consider it as a cause of death in marine animals?

There is a clean-living movement that minimises toxic chemicals in the home. They use bicarbonate of soda and white spirit vinegar to clean. They use no sprays or manufactured products. We forget that it has always been possible to clean this way, and it is only since WW2 that all these toxic chemicals have been available. It is a shame to bring children up in such an environment. Doctors tell us that it is a clean house that damages their immune systems. I would say it is the toxic chemicals we use to do the cleaning that does so.

It is possible to filter the air in your house with plants; but it is better to remove the cause.

It is also possible to make your own toothpaste to avoid fluoride and chemicals, by using one tablespoon of bicarbonate of soda, one tablespoon of xylitol, one tablespoon of coconut oil, and four drops of peppermint essential oil – mixed together thoroughly. Used on a dry toothbrush, it will not damage the biome in your mouth. Fluoride is a toxic additive in toothpaste to try to reduce the amount of decay in children's teeth. In fact, sugar is the cause of the decay, and both children and adults use fluoridated toothpaste. If you have cancer or a chronic disease, you are not tested to see if fluoride is responsible. Usually, doctors say they do not know what causes cancer and chronic disease. The CRUK website lists all the research that they do, but there is no one asking the question: 'Why has this person got this disease at this point in their life?'

Anti-microbial products for hand-cleansing work no better than regular soap and water.

Other Toxic Products

Parfum is not the only problem. Anything that is inhaled, eaten, or put on the skin gets into the body. This includes smells from paint, nail varnish, new furniture, carpets, and clothes. Always wash clothes before wearing them.

Tattoo ink also contains toxic products which end up in the local glands under the arm or in the groin.

Vaping fluid: The main ingredient is propylene glycol (anti-freeze). It also contains vegetable glycerine, nicotine, and natural flavourings like vanilla or sucralose. It damages the cells lining the airways when inhaled, and makes the smoker more liable to infections like streptococcus pneumoniae. Inhaling any chemicals into the lungs should be regarded with suspicion.

Aftershave: It is tempting to use this product to make yourself more attractive (if you believe the adverts), especially if it was bought as a present. But beware if there are any asthmatics in the house.

Mouthwash: They are designed to rid the mouth of the bacteria which cause tooth decay. In fact, they cannot tell which bacteria do which job, so it indiscriminately kills all bacteria. If you keep using it as the manufacturers would have you do, your bacteria will become resistant and you will wreck the biome in your mouth. If you swallow any of it you are absorbing toxic chemicals.

Sunscreens are a real problem. They contain a lot of chemicals to prevent the sun's rays getting through to the skin and causing damage and skin cancer. On the other hand, we need the sun to make vitamin D, which prevents osteoporosis and cancer.

Skin cancer is mainly two types, firstly malignant melanoma, which is difficult to treat and presumably the reason people are advised to protect their skin; although I have seen a 38-year-old patient with one in her bowel, where the sun never reaches. The other types are surface cancers in older people called basal cell and squamous cell, which can easily be removed and rarely spread. So do we trade-off possible prevention of skin damage using toxic chemicals for loss of vitamin D? Why do we not just cover up and wear hats instead? Why do we not just sunbathe for short spells, increasing the time we expose our skin daily? Is the sun the only cause of skin cancer? What about diet, stress, and toxins as well? Could sunscreens be a background cause in the considerable increase in childhood cancers, directly via toxic chemicals or indirectly by preventing the manufacture of vitamin D? The conventional wisdom on the Cancer Research UK website is to use sunscreens all the time, but there is no comment about their efficacy and chemical content, which is considerable.

Sun damage causes ageing, dark marks and discolouration due to melanin pigmentation, and small areas of thickened, darker skin. There are two types of sunscreen – chemical and mineral. Chemical screens contain oxy- and avo-benzones to absorb harmful rays. Mineral screens use physical blockers such as zinc or titanium dioxide.

Household cleaners, often in spray formulation, contain chemicals which are easily inhaled and absorbed through the skin. Instead, it is worth seeing how you get on with bicarbonate of soda and white spirit vinegar – cheap, and effective.

Once again, your liver has to detox all these chemicals and they are excreted via the bile, through to the gut, where they affect the biome. There is not much chance of us all living to 100, never mind 120, when we ingest so many toxins. The older generation were not so badly affected by these products, as they were put on the market after they were grown up.

Noise Pollution

Noise is someone else's sounds. Your sounds are not noise to you. Manmade noise is interpreted by the brain as a danger signal and triggers the stress response. This is why other people's noise makes people angry.

Silence is difficult for most anxious people, but you should end your day with a silent time. Learning yoga and meditation calm the mind.

Being near noise sources puts the blood pressure up due to suppressed anger at not being able to control it.

There has been a Noise Abatement Society since 1959 – recognising the harmful effects of noise on health.

Loud, continuous noise causes deafness, as the auditory nerve shuts down from overstimulation. This is common in people who listen to, or play, loud music, or operate heavy machinery without ear defenders, but it is rare in orchestral players.

Space Junk

Our pollution of the planet is not confined to the Earth. There are millions of pieces of space junk as a result of satellites no longer functioning whilst still orbiting the Earth. This is an important challenge. How do you dispose of satellites no longer needed? If you try to blast them they end up in small pieces rather than bigger ones. Could you manage without your SatNav? When a company needs to send another satellite up to replace an out-of-date one, will there be room? Will they be able to sell you updates if the satellites are not reliable?

Tap Water

It is thanks to reliable tap water that we no longer have to contend with epidemics like cholera, but legionnaires' disease and pseudomonas pneumonia can now be picked up from showers.

However, there is a trade-off. We might not have epidemics of cholera, but tap water now contains drugs that people excrete, and which are not removed before the water is recycled. The main problem is chemical oestrogens from hormone treatment, and cow oestrogen from dairy products. Men are developing breasts, and the incidence of breast and prostate cancer is increasing.

There is also aluminium, fluorine, chlorine, and nitrates in our drinking water. Consequently, some people filter their water. Jug filters remove chlorine and organic compounds, bacteria, and lead, but also magnesium and calcium. Reverse osmosis removes asbestos, bacteria, viruses, fluoride, oestrogen and lead. Bottled water from spring sources is better, but you then have the problem of the chemicals from the plastic bottle leaching into the water.

Additives

Additives are put into food for colouring and to extend the shelf life, and are well known for causing children to run around madly and be generally uncontrollable. Fortunately, the manufacturers removed the offending E-numbers, and this behaviour was alleviated.

Packaging

Plastic is not biodegradable and it mostly ends up in town tips where it stays for centuries, or in the oceans, where it harms fish who eat it.

Antibiotic Residues

These are found in animals reared for meat. As the animals are managed in large numbers they are given antibiotics to prevent disease. Animals that have just had antibiotics are not allowed into the food chain, but that doesn't mean there is none left in the carcass when it is finally slaughtered. They may also be given growth hormones which help them to mature more quickly. Farmers can use homeopathy for this problem, which is cheaper, and ends up with healthier animals.

Toxins From Agriculture

Intensive farming methods need weed killers and pest-controllers to get enough from the land for profit. These have been linked with reduction in the bee pollinators in the area. Cotton production for clothes uses 25% of the world's insecticides.

Plastic Beads

More than 80% of our clothes are made from plastic and we discard one million tons a year. 50% of discarded clothes end up in landfills. Again, plastic does not degrade. The industry is huge, and fills container ships across the world. When you wash your clothes the garments release thousands of plastic fibres into waterways and seas. These fibres, along with the plastic beads from cosmetics, are too small to be filtered by the sewerage system, so end up in the environment and kill any species that ingests them. There is no testing for these particles in humans to see their relationship to disease.

Chemical Sensitivity

Research shows British women come into contact with 680 chemicals of concern on average, each month. They are in toiletries, cosmetics, detergents, cleaners... Is it any wonder the in-home environment has been shown to be more toxic than that of a factory? In 2015, these 'environmental toxins' were shown to link to increased risk of cardiovascular disease, heart attacks, and strokes.

A Royal Commission in the UK warned of 4,000 chemicals of concern in everyday products – saying most were probably toxic, and many were likely carcinogenic!

In 2016 Johnson & Johnson was fined $72 million by a US court over links between talcum powder and ovarian cancer.

But it is largely a history of stalling and inaction. J & J pledged, in August 2012, to eliminate formaldehyde, parabens, triclosan, and phthalates – by 2015 – from all baby products. For adult products, it has removed triclosan and phthalates, but will keep using three parabens, and use formaldehyde in exceptional cases where other preservatives won't work, according to the company's new policy. Who would want to use these chemicals on a baby's skin, and how can the manufacturers sell them as safe for young children?

In 2013 the World Health Organization told world governments they should ban hormone disrupters like parabens, BPA, and phthalates. And in July 2013, triclosan was shown to cause muscle damage that could affect the heart. Always read the ingredients lists, and do not buy anything that contains these chemicals. It is easy to source non-toxic alternatives.

Although the doses in each product may be minimal, xenoestrogens have been shown to be cumulative, so there are really no safe limits. Euro MPs have already voted to remove 1,000 or more chemicals of concern and replace them with safer alternatives. A non-elected commissioner vetoed the decision and set up the REACH project; this may take 15 years at least to complete.

1. Toothpaste contains saccharine, which is an artificial sweetener, fluoride, artificial colours and flavourings, propylene glycol (cosmetic form of mineral oil used in industrial anti-freeze), PEG ingredients, sodium lauryl sulphate (SLS), sodium lauryl ether sulphate (SLES), and triclosan (absorption through the skin can lead to liver damage).

The quickest way into the bloodstream and brain is through the lining of the mouth! What do these chemicals do to the brain? Should CRUK research this sort of issue? Might it have some bearing on the increase in brain tumours in young people?

2. Deodorants and antiperspirants contain formaldehyde, which has caused lung cancer in rats and can damage DNA (it is banned in Japan and Sweden), aluminium, which is linked to cancer and Alzheimer's disease, propylene glycol, parfum, alcohol, triclosan, and parabens. Buy these products, but without the chemicals.

3. Shampoo and conditioner contain formaldehyde (quaternium), PEG, parfum (95% of the chemicals in perfume are synthetic compounds derived from petroleum – 26 of which are on an EU avoidance list), artificial colours, lanolin oil, propylene glycol, BHT, alcohol, isopropanol, paraffin (mineral oil), TEA, MEA, SLS, SLES (these can all lead to potentially carcinogenic cocktails of nitrites and dioxins, which form by reacting with other ingredients), and cocamidopropyl betaine. They are both available without these chemicals in them!

4. Shaving products contain propylene glycol, PEG ingredients, DEA, paraffin, 'eth' ingredients, TEA, MEA, SLS, SLES, benzophenone-3, parabens, and glycerin.

5. Lipstick can contain mineral oil, petrolatum, parfum, lanolin, butylated hydroxyanisole (BHA), titanium dioxide, padimate O, polyethylene, oxybenzone, and

polyvinyl pyrrolidone (PVP). Reports suggest that PVP may cause tumours, and that inhaling its particles could be harmful.

6. Shower gel / liquid soaps can contain sodium lauryl sulfate (SLS), sodium lauryl ether sulfate (SLES), proplylene glycol, PEG ingredients, quaternium, alcohol, artificial colours, fragrance, DEA, TEA, MEA, triclosan, parabens, and glycerin.

7. Foundation contains talc, titanium dioxide, quaternium (formaldehyde), artificial colours, PEG ingredients, propylene glycol (cosmetic form of mineral oil), silica (may be contaminated with cystalline quartz, which is carcinogenic), fragrance, diazolidinyl urea, parabens, and glycerin. Foundation is the most dangerous thing in your make-up bag.

8. Hair spray contains fragrance, alcohol, methylene chloride, toluene, and ether.

9. Hair dyes contain phenylenediamine, which can cause blindness on eye contact, coal tars, hydroxyanisole (which affects the female reproductive system), paraffinum

Iiquidum (mineral oil), fragrance, quaternium, PEG ingredients, 'eth' ingredients, and glycerin. Various medical reports have linked prolonged use of some dark hair dyes to bladder cancer, multiple myeloma, non-Hodgkin's lymphoma, ovarian cancer, and leukaemia.

10. Mouthwash often contains alcohol (mouthwashes with an alcohol content of more than 25% have been linked to mouth, tongue, oesophageal, and throat cancers), fluoride, PEG ingredients, and artificial colours.

11. Nail varnish contains formaldehyde, isopropanol, acetone, acetonitrile (which forms cyanide if swallowed), ethyl, methyl methacrylate, and toluene (methylbenzene/ phenylmethane – a neurotoxin which can damage the liver, disrupt the endocrine system, and cause asthma). Breathing high levels during pregnancy can result in children with birth defects.

12. Talcum and baby powder can contain fragrance and propylene glycol. Talcum powder is linked to the increase in ovarian cancer. It blocks the pores when used in make-up, and may be dangerous when inhaled.

13. Phthalates do not appear on ingredients lists, but are hormone disrupters, and can be leached from plastic bottles, especially if the plastic has been heated (for example, a suncream bottle left in the sun, or a water bottle left in a hot car). Animal studies have shown they can damage the liver, kidneys, lungs, and reproductive system.

The list of chemicals used in the manufacture of household products is worrying. However, there is a choice. It is possible to live without all of these products, as people did before the war.

14. Others include:

Parabens – chemicals which are put into products to extend their shelf lives. They have been identified in breast-cancer tissue and are often found in deodorants.

Sodium laureth sulphate – a chemical included in a formula to produce foaming.

Polyethylene glycol and polystyrene – biosolids which are impossible to remove from the environment and are toxic in the water supply and if ingested.

Formaldehyde and acetaldehyde – class-A carcinogens. They are VOCs, and have been known to cause cancer in humans since the 1980s. They are also produced by cooking, toasters, smoking, heating, consumer products, pressed-wood furniture and laminate floors, and building materials.

Limonene – it produces a citrus smell and is extracted from lemons and oranges. It is found in air fresheners and candles. When exposed to ozone in houses, it is converted to formaldehyde.

Improving Air Quality

We need to know what the problem is that is making us ill before we can do anything about it. Your doctor, GP or specialist is unlikely to be able to advise you, so you need to sort it out yourself.

Ten Tips:

1. Avoid what you can. Get rid of synthetic fragrances.

2. Fifteen to eighteen plants in the house or office will cope with neutralising VOCs. Sick building syndrome includes sleepiness and headaches, and dry eyes can be

helped. Best plants are spider plants, aspidistra, bamboo, fig, and ivy.

3. Homes are built to be airtight, so some ventilation is needed. Heat-recovery ventilation systems are most effective, as they draw in a continuous supply of fresh, filtered air. They are expensive, but can filter out pollen and diesel.

4. Replace thick carpets. House dust contains a cocktail of up to 45 chemicals.

5. Use clay-based paints. Vinyl-based contain VOCs.

6. Vacuum bedrooms twice a week to get rid of house dust mites, as their droppings can cause allergic reactions every day, especially if there are people with asthma in the house. Get rid of carpets and lay linoleum instead.

7. Eliminate black mould. Scrub with vinegar and borax substitute, and ensure good ventilation.

8. Make your own natural cleaners. Use bicarbonate and vinegar. You will find they work just as well. If you want fragrances use natural oils like lavender, which can be applied with a small spray bottle.

9. If you have a wood-burning stove, maintain it regularly. Clean the flue annually, check the door seal is working properly, and only burn seasoned wood. Send smokers outside.

10. Invest in an indoor air-pollution monitor. This kit measures VOCs and diesel, and costs about £130.

11. Charcoal is good at absorbing pollutants and can be found in cosmetics to use on the skin, and in toothpaste.

Wi-Fi

Wi-Fi is an electromagnetic frequency. It has the ability to break DNA chains, causing alterations in the blood-brain barrier, and can disrupt brain glucose metabolism, as well as cell metabolism.

This can cause symptoms of fatigue, irritability, headaches, and digestive disorders.

Long-term exposure is linked to the breaking up of single- and double-stranded DNA, with memory loss, diabetes, depression, insomnia, and cancers resulting.

Solutions are:

1. Avoid using Wi-Fi in a vehicle because of increased exposure when the frequencies are bounced around.

2. Turn Wi-Fi off when not in use, especially at night.

3. Use an Ethernet system at home, which is hardwired.

4. Keep the Wi-Fi source as far away as possible from where you sit at home.

5. Suggest that your neighbours do the same.

9

GENES, CANCER, AND SLOW VIRUSES

When I started in general practice I came equipped with a diploma in family planning, so I asked my partners if I could start a clinic in the practice. I had been taught about following up patients in gynaecological practice, carrying out smears on them all. As a student we had been expected to do smears on all gynaecological patients, as there was a good pathology service set up in Newcastle and Gateshead to read them. This was not long after the Pap smear had been introduced. I therefore asked my partners about this as well. They agreed that it was a good thing to offer patients but they had had no training in it, so it was left to me to organise the system.

It was a great success. After a while I became concerned about the number of patients with infections reported by the lab. The infections had not always been obvious on examination. I talked to the bacteriologist about this and said I thought I ought to know if patients had hidden infections, and asked if I could swab them and see what was wrong. She agreed that I could do a small survey of 25 consecutive patients who had infections on their smear reports. The ones with abnormal cells were referred to a gynaecologist in the usual way, but there were none in my group of 25.

To our surprise they all had infections: out of 25 patients, 3 had chlamydia, 18 had candida (thrush), and the rest had viral infections and bacterial vaginosis. There were no sexually transmitted diseases and the viruses were not identified. They were all treated – chlamydia and bacterial vaginosis with antibiotics, thrush with anti-fungals, and the viral infections with iodine pessaries. When the smears were repeated they were all clear. This was a big lesson to me that women harbour viruses in their cervix, and they are left to simmer and were never recognised nor treated.

What effect do viruses have, which are not the ones that cause cancer of the cervix (HPV, the human papillomavirus), if they sit there for years? Are they transmissible to babies as they are being born? It seemed like a missed opportunity not to sort this problem out for women, as we do not know what we might be able to prevent. It is *still* a missed opportunity, as nurses now do smears without the ability to diagnose and treat obvious infections. Only the patients with abnormal cells are referred. Some viruses would be leaking into the bloodstream, and the immune system is continually stressed by this. I also realised that the number of people with thrush needed an explanation.

As we have already seen, the consequences of abnormal bacteria in the gut is far-reaching and contributes considerably to the development of disease. Genes are turned on and off by psycho-neuro-hormono-immunology, and an abnormal biome.

When you become infected, for example with a cold, your immune system responds by causing inflammation in your respiratory tract. Hopefully this causes complete eradication of the infecting organism, but if it does not then viruses are left in your system. They are mostly in your gut, including the appendix, pancreas and gallbladder. From time to time they escape into the circulation and may lodge in the brain, arterial walls, uterus, pancreas, or in fact any organ. Any cell with a virus in it will react to try to eradicate it. If the cell is overstimulated and this causes sequences of genes to be switched on or off, then it may turn into a cancerous cell. If it is unable to respond, it dies. The response needs to be exact to cope, as Darwin discovered. *The survival of the*

289

fittest! If your immune system does not work properly, you will not survive to reproduce and pass your genes on as they are faulty. This is how children have acquired lifelong immunity to measles, etc. Their immune systems were triggered to respond appropriately to the infection, as a result of thousands of years of practise.

Cancer

Between 200 and 1,000 precancerous cells are produced in the body daily. The immune system detects and deals with them. The mitochondria in the cells power them and allow the cells to take in carbohydrates and oxygen to make energy.

To make a cancerous cell there will be genetic changes to the DNA and mitochondria, plus a variety of other factors. These factors, like nutrition and diet, may well be variable for each person. The mitochondria no longer work properly and do not use oxygen. In fact, oxygen can kill cancer cells. Oestrogen makes cancer cells proliferate. Oestrogen decreases folic acid (a B vitamin) in the body, which is needed to copy DNA/RNA correctly. When levels are low mistakes are made and cancer cells are produced. This is why folic acid is so important in pregnancy for the growing foetus, to prevent mistakes in the developing cells. Oestrogen can also help cancer spread and makes cells proliferate.

As reported in the last chapter, a lot of household chemicals can mimic oestrogen – mainly parfum in detergents and cosmetics. Cow oestrogen also affects cancer cell growth as a result of eating dairy products.

The 'Never Well Since' Syndrome

When there were a lot of childhood infections about, there were some children who developed long-term consequences. Whooping cough could cause winter bronchitis. Recurrent bronchitis causes damage to the lungs over many years, and in one of my patients, bronchiectasis – damaged, dilated alveoli. The only treatment offered was antibiotics, inhalers, steroids, and surgery. She regularly had lobes of the left lung removed, until she only had one lung left. Two years later the bronchiectasis started in the remaining lung. She had regular homeopathic treatment in general practice from me, and antibiotics from my partners. Her consultants were surprised at how long it took for the bronchiectasis to reappear in the right lung (over two years). They never asked why.

We recognise this syndrome in homeopathy as the 'never well since' syndrome, but I've never heard it expressed in this way by conventional medicine, as there is no concept of it. It would not help diagnosis or treatment. Your past medical history seems to be much less important now than it used to be. In fact, our previous history may be deleted from the computer in the surgery after ten years or so, as it is not deemed relevant after that amount of time.

It is also expressed by patients saying that since they had glandular fever, flu, or gastroenteritis, they have not really recovered and feel tired all the time. What it usually indicates is that the patient was under stress before the illness struck, and their poor immune system has not been able to cope with the infection and has left them exhausted. It is therefore the stress that causes the problem and must be resolved, but is rarely asked about by doctors.

Slow Viruses and Bacteria

The idea of slow viruses does not seem to be a concept in conventional medicine at the present time. However, when infectious diseases were common, people knew that certain viruses had affinity for certain organs, like mumps in the pancreas and testicles. Herpes viruses are always associated with the nervous system, and many others with the gut, gallbladder and liver. If the virus sits in these tissues for many years and the patient is stressed, which causes a decrease in the functioning of the immune system, it is possible that the viruses will trigger a cancerous response. Vets know that feline leukaemia is caused by a virus, so why should this not be so in humans?

An example of acute and chronic or slow infections is shown by the streptococcus bacteria. Acute infections cause tonsillitis and scarlet fever. If the streptococcus is not totally eliminated, the toxin ends up in different parts of the brain and causes Tourette's syndrome. I treated an eight year old with Tourette's with the homeopathic remedy belladonna. At the second consultation he was improving. His mum told me about research that showed the streptococcal toxin in areas of the brain as the cause of the symptoms, so I also gave him the remedy streptococcin, made from the streptococcus group. She also showed me a copy of a ten-page document written by a clinical psychologist about his behaviour, who wrote that there was nothing of any note in his history, but did not see the significance of his repeated attacks of tonsillitis as a small child and his mother's history of streptococcal infection after his birth. My patient was considerably improved after the homeopathic treatment. His consultant invited me to go and talk to him, which I did. He was very impressed, but said it was no help to him in the long run, as he was not in a position to learn the discipline of homeopathy.

There always used to be an increase in type 1 diabetes in children after a mumps epidemic, because the mumps virus settled in the pancreas with slow destruction of the cells that produce insulin. Other viruses in the pancreas associated with type 1 diabetes are coxsackie B, rotavirus and cytomegalovirus. A virus infection in the gut may settle in the pancreas and cause inflammation, and an immune response in the islet cells that produce insulin. If the inflammation results in scarring there is deficiency of insulin. Where does the modified virus in the mumps vaccine end up? Does it have any relevance to the vast number of diabetics in the world, and does it account for the increase in pancreatic cancer?

It may not be the correct thing to do to prevent illness by vaccination if your immune system is designed to be educated (programmed) to deal with invaders and inflammation by being frequently exposed to these events over your life.

Viruses causing cancer were first researched in the 1930s. The research showed that:

1. Chicken sarcomas could be transmitted to healthy chickens by injections from the affected one.

2. In 1936 a mouse mammary tumour virus was discovered, which also could be transmitted to healthy mice by injection of the affected tissue.

3. More recently, other viruses were discovered that cause cancers, like the hepatitis virus, which causes Kaposi's sarcoma, and the human T-cell lymphotropic virus, which causes Burkitt's lymphoma in African children.

4. A single gene called the SRC gene in a virus may be responsible for cancer. A wide range of animals carry this

gene in their DNA. If the SRC gene becomes faulty it turns cancerous.

5. Feline leukaemia is caused by a retrovirus that 2% of cats carry. It is the commonest cause of cancer in cats. It may be years between the cat acquiring the virus and the cancer developing. Similarly, human leukaemia is usually acute in children and chronic in adults.

When a virus invades a human, if the immune system is effective, the patient recovers. If the immune system is overwhelmed and cannot respond, the patient may die. If the immune system copes partially, the patient may be left with obvious damage – like brain damage from measles – or without damage, but with circulating viruses left dormant, possibly in the bone marrow.

Why has there been such a huge increase in cancers in children, teenagers and young adults? Cancer used to be a disease of old age.

Cancer Research UK says you can't catch cancer but you obviously can catch the invaders that are associated with it. It also says that having certain pathogens in various sites in the body increases the risk of cancer. Like H. pylori in cancer of the stomach, the Epstein-Barr virus in

Hodgkin's lymphoma, and HIV and sarcoma. In other countries liver worms cause bile-duct cancer, although I had an English patient with this cancer, and Schistosoma, a river worm in Africa, causes bladder cancer.

The point is, that it's not the virus that causes the cancer, it is the psycho-neuro-hormono-immunology behind it. Would you get the cancer if you had the virus but not the background affecting you? Probably not, because your immune system would not turn the genes on or off to allow the cancer to develop.

CRUK spends a lot of money finding a way of getting virus parts that are non-pathogenic into cells to carry medication directly to the cancer. It is one of the few ways modern medicine can cope with treating cancer, as the pathway via P-N-H-I is too difficult. This is why people look to homeopathy for treatment for the whole person with cancer, and not just for the cancer alone.

So it would appear that viruses are important in causing disease a long time after they originally invaded the body. It seems odd that they are not included in the NHS list which says that risk factors for lung cancer are cigarette smoke, radon gas, asbestos, uranium, inhaled chemicals like arsenic, beryllium, cadmium, silica, vinyl, nickel, chromium, coal products, mustard gas in WW1, chloromethyl ether, diesel exhaust fumes, household cleaners, and smoking marijuana and radiation therapy for cancers (treat with one hand and cause with the other). If it is known that household cleaners are a risk for cancer, why are the chemicals not removed, or a warning put on the containers?

Viruses are linked to 40% of cancers:

1. Cytomegalovirus (which causes a glandular-fever-like illness), to childhood brain cancers;

2. Hepatitis B and C, to liver cancer;

3. Merkel cell polyomavirus, to the skin cancer melanoma;

4. The Epstein-Barr virus (glandular fever), to blood and lymph cancers;

5. The human papillomavirus is commonly found in prostate cancer, as it is in cervical cancer.

Why do oncologists not look for viruses? They say that it could be one of many viruses in prostate cancer, but what is the virus in a particular patient? They say it would be no help to identify a virus as there is no medication for viruses, so chemotherapy and radiation therapy are used instead. In homeopathy there is always treatment for viral infections.

As far as cancer development is concerned, you can live a very healthy lifestyle, but it is your anxiety levels that count eventually, which is why so few people will live to be 120, and genetics will never be an answer to this problem. It is never bad luck which causes cancer. If doctors say this, it means they do not understand or they feel you are not up to a rational discussion. It is *always* things in your life which cause cancer.

Genes

Genes are the instructions for making all parts of the human body and brain. They are made up of DNA and packaged onto strands called chromosomes. We have two copies of all our genes, so our chromosomes are in pairs.

We all know that we have a completely individual set of genes that make us different to each other. They respond to environmental factors and it is not possible to have any disease without genes being switched, and they must be switched in the correct sequence. This mechanism may well be learnt by the body throughout life in response to childhood infections, etc. Now children are vaccinated, this response may not be learnt.

Studies of genetically identical twins show that both develop different diseases over the course of their lives. If you are identified as carrying the gene for a specific condition, you may not get it if the circumstances to switch the gene sequence on or off don't occur. Gene behaviour is never simple. They cascade, interact, dance, and generally refuse to behave anything like a computer, despite being made of four bases that look a lot like computer code. It is not merely the existence and location of genes that matter, but their complicated interactions and control systems. Your biome regulates homoeostasis, and there are direct connections between your biome and epigenetic gene regulation.

Gene Therapy

In the 1980s it was postulated that if you found the gene that causes an illness (like cystic fibrosis), and if it is missing or damaged, it could be replaced and good health would ensue. Unfortunately this theory failed when trialled, and deaths occurred. Recently it has been suggested that if you find such a gene in a foetus, for example, for Huntington's chorea, there is a choice to abort or alter in the womb. It is not known what makes your genes healthy and unable to be switched on or off, or stay switched to cause disease. It is not known what activates your genes. It is also not known what micronutrients are needed in this process. The only reason for finding out why and how the gene cascade works other than pure science is to find some medication to alter it. However, it is thought that this is one of the ways homeopathic medicines work – by switching genes on or off during disease.

It is probable in due course that every child at birth will have its genome, the totality of its genes, mapped. They will then know what diseases are likely to develop and what precautions might be taken for prevention. This supposes that everyone will be prepared to take advice and carry it out. It hasn't happened with smoking, drugs, alcohol, etc. People always think that it will never happen to them. It is very difficult for most of the population to translate advice given to them as a percentage risk in their own life.

The sequencing of the human genome was completed in 2003, and it was assumed that it was then going to be easy to cure, prevent and eradicate all disease. It has not happened so far as it has raised more questions than answers. Trying to alter DNA proved difficult if not dangerous. Several deaths occurred in trials. The main problem has been that we didn't have the tools to cut minute lengths of genes, and even the smallest mistake can have far-reaching effects. Now viruses called bacteriophages are used to separate sequences of DNA with amazing accuracy. Genetic engineering has become editing. The question is what we can, should, and will do with the knowledge. So far it has mainly been used in plants and animals, and produces tomatoes that never rot and mosquitos incapable of transmitting malaria, which are then released and produce generations of mosquitos that are not able to carry the disease. This technique, called CRISPR, has been used to cure mice of cataracts and muscular dystrophy, but such treatments are not likely to be used in humans for some years.

If you have your DNA sequenced, you may be able to find out what sort of diet you should eat to keep you slim and healthy. There is a number of companies online that offer this service.

302

Certain genes raise the risk of dementia and this is the sort of problem that CRISPR may make an impact on. This may also mean that particular genes express anxiety and indirectly switch the genes on for dementia.

Genomics

The study of gene sequencing. When Dame Sally Davies was the Chief Medical Officer, she said that she thought DNA sequencing should be as routine as blood tests and biopsies. The idea is to find the cause of your disease. However, it is not the gene which causes the disease, but the reason why the genes are switched on or off. You cannot have any disease without genes in the background. It all depends on what level of impact it takes to switch them. Dr Davies hoped that the UK would be able to expand its 10% share of the £8 billion global genomics market.

Epigenetics

Epigenetics is the science of finding out how our genes transfer information through the generations and respond to environmental factors like trauma – both physical and mental. It links cancer, heart disease, respiratory disease, and autoimmune disease to the parents' and grandparents' histories and how genes interact or communicate with one another. It is known that life events can change the genetic destiny of future generations and cause disease. Alterations in the genes are caused by poor diet, stress, environmental toxins (VOCs), and hormones like oestrogen. Blockages affect the levels of methionine and homocysteine in the body, which affect methylation on your DNA. There is a build-up of histones around (epi) DNA (genes) and blockages are formed so that messages cannot be read or sent out. It is not a mutation, which is a sequence change in DNA coding.

This is behind all disease: the effect that the environment, mental stress, and physical damage has on our genes.

There have been 17 genes identified for depression, and some depression runs in families. Identifying genes that affect risk for a disease is the first step towards understanding the disease itself. This may provide targets to aim for in developing new treatments if you are interested in drugs, but makes no difference if you use homeopathy as a therapy. It is thought that homeopathic remedies work by telling the brain to signal the switching of genes on or off, which would cure.

Every cell in the body has a nucleus of genes. In the ovary and testes the sperm and ova contain 46 chromosomes and an X and Y chromosome to determine the sex of the child. Each chromosome contains genetic material that gets passed on. Your genetic make-up reflects heredity, how you were brought up, where you live, what you eat, how you used your brain and your emotional and personality development, your job, your income, happiness, and ability to cope. This means that throughout your life your genes are constantly adjusting to what your body experiences. As of now, your genes reflect all that, but along the way they've been altered by things that have happened to you, especially stress.

Genes respond to external factors like smoking, toxic chemicals in your environment, and your biome. If you smoke, you never know if your genes and immune system will support you to a good age, or if you are destined to die early of cancer or heart disease.

Genetic Mutations

Eight different conditions that cause mitochondrial disease, which is a result of genetic mutations, have been identified. They cause a lack of thymidine phosphorylase and therefore DNA is not built properly. This shows itself as a muscle-wasting disease. The function of the mitochondrial DNA in the nuclei of cells is impaired and the cell is unable to convert energy from food into a form that can be used by the cells.

Some genetic diseases are caused by missing genes, as in metabolic disorders like hemochromatosis (iron metabolism) and Wilson's disease (copper metabolism), haemophilia, sickle cell disease, and cystic fibrosis – or too many chromosomes (structures full of genes), as in Down's syndrome.

Many more genetic mutations or absences have been identified, and it would appear that you do not get any condition unless genes are involved.

Behavioural Genetics

Behavioural genetics are methods used to investigate the nature and origins of individual differences in behaviour. It has moved researchers' focus from individual genes to entire genomes. A goal of modern neuroscience is to understand how genes and their expression interact with neuronal network function to produce complex behaviours; in other words, how your genes and brain interact. Variation amongst individuals is separated into genetic versus environmental components. It is most commonly researched using family studies, twin studies, and adoption studies. It looks at aspects of life like anxiety. Are you genetically programmed to be more or less anxious, or do you pick it up from your environment? How much of each is relevant to each person's behaviour?

A goal of modern neuroscience is to understand how genes and their expression interact with neuronal network function to produce complex behaviours.

The way your immune system responds is also genetically programmed, and depends on what has stimulated it during your life.

Viruses, Genes, and Cancer

Diagnoses for cancer are the highest on record, with 822 people diagnosed every day, and a total of 299,923 in 2015.

It would appear that viruses, genes, and cancer are intimately related. HIV, which causes AIDS, has been stripped down to a small portion that enters and reprogrammes cells to hunt down and kill cancer cells. Experimental trials are underway in humans. The virus portion carries treatment directly into the cancer cells. The medication to be carried into cancerous cells is manufactured by a drug company.

Structural Biology

Cancer is enormously complex. It can adapt and evolve as its environment changes, and in response to treatment. The scientists who look at structural biology look at the fundamental mechanisms at work in the development and progression, right down to the smallest level, like how proteins signal to one another. Proteins are required for the structure, function and regulation of nearly everything

308

that happens in our tissues and organs, including the cells' messaging system. In cancer cells this messaging system is defective, which may be due to faulty versions of proteins that can adopt a different shape, or due to incorrect connections between the cells' messengers. Cancer cells exploit such changes to drive their own growth and spread. Biologists are presently studying the three-dimensional structure of proteins to increase their understanding of how they work and communicate.

Immunotherapy

At present, cancer treatment is unsatisfactory. It causes many side effects and there is no guarantee that it will be effective. Recently, one of the drug companies said that a long-awaited lung-cancer treatment had failed to deliver. Its shares tumbled. Their results showed that their immunotherapy treatment did not stop cancer worsening in patients for any longer than existing treatments.

If immunotherapy is used with anticancer drugs, then:

1. 11% achieve quite good results for their cancer treatment.

2. 30% develop diabetes because the major immunotherapeutic medication is steroids.

3. 15% develop autoimmune disease.

4. 2% die in the first two weeks.

5. 42% achieve poor results for their cancer treatment.

Poliomyelitis

This virus infection was last seen in the UK as an epidemic in 1957. That means that it is unlikely that any practicing doctor has seen an acute case. They may have done if they have worked abroad.

Bill Gates has funded a charity to try to eliminate worldwide polio by vaccination. Forty-five million children annually will be given the polio vaccine until 2020, when it is hoped that the world will be polio-free. The UK has pledged a generous amount of money. Polio was wiped out in the UK by the 1980s, but there are still currently 100,000 survivors of the illness from childhood. I treated three patients with post-polio syndrome with homeopathy, and they all had relief from their symptoms.

Wild polio is still seen in Afghanistan, Nigeria and Pakistan, with eight new cases in 2016. Cases of polio and paralysis occurred after the live polio vaccine was given to two million children in Syria – similarly in India. There is also a syndrome called vaccine-associated paralytic polio, which occurs as a side effect to the oral polio vaccine. In fact, the oral vaccine is no longer used in the USA, because it is shed from the bowel into sewers, and sanitation and water systems.

This tends to suggest that the wild poliovirus and its altered form in the vaccine are slow viruses, and may remain in the body forever. If so, it might only take an alteration in stress levels with the inability to cope, the immune system affected, the wrong nutrition, and the switching of genes for it to develop into a neurodegenerative disease. The poliovirus sits in the anterior horn cells of the spinal cord waiting for the circumstances to be right for it to flourish. If it does, it would produce the symptoms of polio, but without the acute onset and fever of the original disease. The comparison with motor neurone disease is identical. The incidence of motor neurone disease is increasing, and five people a day die from it in the UK. In 30 years we had no cases in my practice.

ACUTE POLIO	MOTOR NEURONE DISEASE
1. Acute infection of the anterior horn cells	1. Chronic disease of the anterior horn cells
2. Rare – because of immunisation?	2. Much more common now than when acute polio was around
3. Mild, moderate, and severe with paralysis	3. Unremitting onset of paralysis
4. Paralysis of limbs, swallowing, and breathing	4. Paralysis of limbs, swallowing, and breathing
5. Flaccid paralysis, late contractures, altered sensations, retention of urine	5. Wasting then stiffness, altered sensations, neuralgia, cramps, fasciculation, spasticity, retention of urine
6. Mental confusion, drowsiness, irregular pulse, irregular respiration, dysphagia, paralysis of tongue, palate and facial muscles, difficulty speaking and swallowing, unable to keep the jaw shut	6. Paralysis of facial muscles, tongue, larynx, pharynx, difficulty speaking and swallowing, unable to keep the jaw shut

The similarities between acute polio and motor neurone disease are obvious from the table above. If this is so, why do neurologists not consider this diagnosis for patients with MND? The problem is that it would not help, as it would make no difference to the management of the patient. There is no medication. However, there is a polio nosode in homeopathy which would be well worth using, as it helped considerably with the patients I treated with post-polio syndrome.

10

REWIRING THE BRAIN:
Autism, ADHD, PTSD, and Cancer

We have seen that shocks can alter the brain. They can also be the origin of severe anxiety. What if shocks also rewire the brain to cause other diseases? The outcome of severe shock, that is, a shock that the body cannot cope with, is for the brain to shut down. It may shut down from physical shock, as in a coma as a result of brain injury after an accident, or from mental shock, which is terror. Terror affects the whole body via psycho-neuro-hormono-immunology. The effect is profound. Only parts of the brain shut down. The memory of the event is stored in the hard drive, i.e., the subconscious, and may therefore surface in dreams. Does anyone know what children with autism dream about? An event which causes an acute fear of death is truly life-changing.

The parts of the brain that shut down are different in each person, which is why people with autism have different symptoms. The reason why a part of the brain is affected in different people must be to do with the way the brain

314

has already developed, and consequently some parts will be more able to withstand shock.

Brain shutdown can be expressed in many ways, for example, mutism, paralysis, poor speech, and comprehension, which are physical manifestations, or are consequences of anxiety, like handflapping and tidying up. It is not necessary to be conscious to respond to shock, as people in ICUs also experience it, and they are usually heavily sedated. It is a pity that the ICU consultants in this country do not use the homeopathic remedies aconite, for shock, and arnica, for injury. In countries where they *are* used, the recovery time is significantly shorter and PTSD is less common.

Shock may also be caused by physical assaults from chemicals.

ADHD

Attention deficit hyperactivity disorder is described by NHS Choices as a group of behavioural symptoms that include inattentiveness, hyperactivity, and impulsiveness. Common problems include a short attention span, being easily distracted, restlessness, constant fidgeting, overactivity, and being impulsive. All these symptoms are also symptoms of anxiety.

Causes

According to NHS Choices, factors include genetics, brain function and structure, being born prematurely, having a low birth weight, brain damage (either in the womb or in the first few years of life), high maternal alcohol intake, smoking or taking recreational drugs while pregnant, and exposure to high levels of toxic lead at a young age. In fact, these are not causes but statistical risk factors, all of them able to cause shock to the foetus.

The epidemic rise of this condition and the huge number of children who are growing up diagnosed with ADHD suggest that it is more than drug companies profiting from diagnosing 'behaviour' as 'illness', but an actual increase. It is being diagnosed worldwide.

The main problem, especially in the USA, seems to be that children are being diagnosed with ADHD, then prescribed Ritalin for many years as it is the only medication that might help. The choice of medication is interesting, as Ritalin can *cause* behavioural problems in children, so if it works, it seems to be using the homeopathic principle – treating like with like.

There has been a huge increase in ADHD across the globe. Its growth started in the USA some 50 years ago, moved to the UK, Germany, France, Italy, and Brazil. A prodigious rise of drug-based treatment accompanied it. In the UK, ADHD is now the most prevalent behavioural disorder, with an estimated 3.9% of children and adolescents having the condition.

The influence of drug companies, and in the USA psychiatry, which has promoted the use of drugs rather than psychotherapy, has given the drug companies the ability to move into the rest of the world. As the American market became saturated, big pharma expanded into international markets, and promoted ADHD drug treatment around the world, first in Europe, but also in countries such as Brazil, Mexico, and Japan.

Children with ADHD grow up into adults with ADHD, and the market for adults is growing faster than for children and long-acting (16 hours) medication has been developed. Adults now make up more than half the market.

Patient advocacy groups often work closely with drug companies in promoting drug treatments. In some countries, such as France and Italy, ADHD rates are lower, possibly arising from a stronger cultural tradition of using psychological rather than drug-based approaches for behavioural problems, and greater restrictions on the use of ADHD drugs. Even if the diagnosis is between behaviour and disease, it does not matter for homeopathic treatment, because behaviour rather than disease is treated.

There are many factors known or suspected to cause ADHD, all relating to our modern environment.

Chemicals

Damage from:
1. Pesticides, which are widely used to grow the amount of food needed to keep the population fed;
2. Other noxious chemicals, for cleaning and other purposes, used in households;
3. VOCs;

4. Lead, aluminium, mercury and toxic plastic materials.

No one studies what effect their use has in foetal and newborn brains.

Diet

Aspects of our modern diet, particularly highly processed artificial foods and drinks, sugar, artificial sweeteners, food colourings, and additives have frequently been blamed for hyperactivity. It has been suggested that GMO foods might also be implicated.

Conventional Medical Drugs

Anaesthesia: Anaesthesia has been implicated in causing many forms of brain damage, including ADHD. Researchers at the Mayo Clinic compared the records of a group of children exposed to two or more anaesthetics before the age of three, with a group that had had no exposure. It was found that the former group had over twice the incidence of ADHD as the latter. They found that statistically, the data showed a very large difference between each group, and a clear correlation between anaesthesia and cognitive impairment.

Painkillers: Common painkillers, taken by mothers prior to birth, have also been implicated in hyperactivity and behavioural disorders. Paracetamol taken by mothers when pregnant has been associated with ADHD. A study in the USA found that children exposed to paracetamol (acetaminophen) prenatally are at increased risk of multiple behavioural difficulties, and the link was not explained by behavioural or social factors linked to the drug. Around 5% of children developed multiple behavioural problems after their mother had taken the painkiller while pregnant, according to researchers at the University of Bristol. They reviewed 7,796 mothers; 95% had taken paracetamol during pregnancy, and 89% carried on taking the painkiller after the birth. Behavioural problems were reported when the child was checked at the age of five, and again two years later.

It appears that the increase in the rate of ADHD and autism throughout much of the world may be largely mediated by the marked increase in the use of paracetamol in genetically and/or metabolically susceptible children, and the use of paracetamol by pregnant women.

Because many children with ADHD and autism have biochemically defective sulphation, they cannot properly detoxify paracetamol. Therefore, it becomes toxic in the gut. This then leads to intestinal clostridia bacterial overgrowth and a poor biome.

Clostridia bacteria cause overproduction of brain dopamine and reduced concentrations of brain noradrenaline.

Too much dopamine leads to obsessive, compulsive, and stereotypical behaviours.

Too little adrenaline leads to reduced exploratory behaviour and learning in new environments.

Because sulphation is often defective in people with ADHD and autism, the body cannot use proper pathways to get rid of paracetamol. Therefore, the body sends a larger than normal amount of paracetamol to be detoxified by a pathway called cytochrome P450 2E1.

The problem with this pathway is that it leads to excessive production of a very toxic metabolite, which is dangerous because it depletes glutathione and reduces the body's ability to detoxify a host of toxic chemicals from the environment.

In addition, the increase of this toxic metabolite creates oxidative stress which leads to protein, lipid, and nucleic acid damage from free radicals. It also causes an increased rate of damage to mitochondrial and nuclear DNA.

Paracetamol is not the safe painkiller we always were led to believe. It is still given to children for fevers and teething. It would seem to be much safer to try homeopathic remedies instead.

Other risk factors include antidepressant drugs taken whilst pregnant, and amalgam teeth fillings which contain the poison mercury. Vaccines for many years were also manufactured with mercury in the vials to prevent deterioration of the contents.

Vaccines

The drugs most seriously implicated in causing the ADHD and autism epidemics are vaccines – in particular the early childhood vaccines, DPT, MMR, and flu. In the USA it has been found that several vaccines are linked to a range of neuropsychiatric conditions, such as obsessive-compulsive disorder (OCD), ADHD, bipolar, and major depression. It was suspected that vaccines, flu in particular, were affecting the immune system, which influences brain development. All the problems could be categorised as iatrogenic autoimmune disorders.

Unfortunately, it is these links between profitable pharmaceutical drugs and disease that are the most resisted by the conventional medical establishment, supported by a compliant mainstream media.

Yet the evidence supporting the link between vaccines and mental illnesses, including ADHD, is extremely strong, and an Internet search will reveal a lot of information.

Autism

The care of people with autism is now big business, and growing. In every London borough, 300 new children a year are being diagnosed with autism. As students, we were shown the only known case in the 1,000 Families Study, as the condition was so rare.

Autism is much more common in boys and this is thought to be because boys have a less mature immune system at birth. It is a worldwide phenomenon and has increased dramatically since the 1980s. One in a hundred people in the UK is affected. The rate seems to be increasing by 10% annually. It occurs most commonly in developed countries. Vets also find it in cats and dogs.

My interest in autism was fuelled by attending a seminar about the homeopathic treatment of autism. The speaker told us about Dr Tinus Smits, a Dutch homeopathic doctor who was threatened with a court case because he had apparently claimed to have cured 300 children of autism. When it turned out that it was not Dr Smits who was claiming the cures, but the children's mothers, the case against him was dropped. It had been brought by big pharma.

However, he had done a lot of research and had come up with a list of causes. The research was easy to do. He just asked the parents what they thought had happened.

Dr Smits came up with over 40 causes, all of which had something in common: they had caused the baby to suffer shock. Shock, as we have seen, is very important in causing disease, as it rewires the brain. On Dr Smits' website there is a video taken by a parent of a child the day before and the day after their vaccination. The difference is appalling. Beforehand, the baby was acting quite normally. Afterwards, it was pale, indifferent, and not eating. The baby took weeks to recover its senses and emerged damaged and with autism.

His homeopathic treatment cured the children of all their varied symptoms, from handflapping, body-spinning, headbanging, food intolerances, agitation, hyperactivity, recurrent colds, fevers and asthma, stomach pains, constipation/diarrhoea, and failure to grow and thrive – but not learning disability, as if that part of the brain was permanently shut down.

Adults with autism are usually infertile, not sexually active, and die younger than they should, often from heart disease or suicide.

Asperger's syndrome is a version of autism where the patient rarely has learning difficulty, and in fact may be exceptionally clever. They can be very superstitious and obsessed with colours. It is known that a lot of people with this condition are employed at GCHQ because they are good at puzzles and maths.

Symptoms of Autism

Each child or adult is different, but common features are:

- Delayed or unusual speech patterns

- Fits

- Learning disabilities

- Lack of eye contact

- Hypersensitivity, or hyposensitivity, to light, sounds, touch, and crowds

- Repetitive behaviour such as handflapping, tidying, and rotating their body

- Poor verbal interaction or mutism

- Gastrointestinal problems like lactose and gluten intolerances, with symptoms of diarrhoea and constipation

- Severe anxiety, for which the repetitive movements, for example, can act as a comforting mechanism

Autism Toxicity Checklist

Dr Smits' list from the parents' questionnaires:

Before Pregnancy:

In the father and mother, possibly invoking genetic memory, or leaving a permanent disturbance.

1. Tropical vaccinations: DPT, typhoid, yellow fever, hepatitis A and B, cholera, rabies

2. Malaria-prevention medication

3. Illnesses like glandular fever, Lyme disease, hepatitis B, colitis, asthma, epilepsy, migraines, and the medication taken for them, especially antibiotics and steroids

4. Anaesthesia and surgery

5. Dental treatment with amalgam fillings

6. Tetanus vaccine after injury

7. IVF and the drugs to produce ova

8. Contraceptive pills

9. Use of creams with steroids

10. Botox and implants

11. Tattoos

12. Use of recreational drugs

During Pregnancy:

1. Vaccines

2. Medication of ANY sort for acute or chronic illness

3. Dental treatment with amalgam fillings

4. Antibiotics

5. Artificial sweeteners

6. Paracetamol 500 mg, which also contains aspartame

7. Medication during labour, like injections for inhibiting contractions in premature labour (steroids), injections for maturing lungs in a premature baby, and pain relief

8. Household toxins like deodorants, containing parfum and aluminium, mostly used as a spray

9. Medication for constipation, like liquorice

10. Strong emotional events

11. Smoking and alcohol

12. Use of recreational drugs

13. Pre-eclamptic toxaemia

14. Threatened miscarriage

During Delivery:

1. Medication to stimulate contractions or delay the onset of early labour

2. Any medication including anaesthetics and analgesics

3. Obstructed labour with foetal distress and/or a poor Apgar score

4. Cord around neck

5. Caesarean section

First Two Years of Life – and if Breastfed:

1. All vaccinations

2. All medication given to baby or mother

3. Anaesthetics, especially for grommets

4. Plastic feeding bottles warmed up in a microwave, plastic dummies, vinyl in the bedroom, soft plastics in contact with food

5. Investigations with contrast agents

6. Circumcision

The outcome of all these insults is a shock to the baby. The baby's brain responds by shutting down because it cannot cope. When it does recover it rewires, but differently, which accounts for the unusual symptoms. It is a version of brain damage or post-traumatic stress disorder. Harm to the brain-gut connection via the vagus nerve accounts for damage to the biome, and the symptoms of diarrhoea and food intolerances. It leaves the child extremely anxious, with a poor immune system.

Treatment

Everyone knows that autism is a lifelong, incurable condition. The only aspect of the symptoms that can be managed by doctors is to avoid the foods causing gut problems, if they have been diagnosed. The usual first step is to refer for speech therapy.

The brain-gut connection in autism has been known about since a mother in the USA asked her gastroenterologist to investigate her son's diarrhoea. The first thing he found was a low level of the pancreatic hormone secretin. So from then on, he gave children injections of secretin and they improved mentally, as well as their diarrhoea improving, reflecting the connection between brain and body. Unfortunately, the effect of the injected secretin was not long-lived in the body and so more and more injections were needed. It was not a practical solution, but showed how important gut function is in this condition.

The Sunderland University website for autism asked parents to say what had helped their children, and they mainly reported a gluten- and/or lactose-free diet, which seemed to be evidence of parents knowing what was going on in their children, but doctors not listening.

Autistic children can be extremely anxious, and their behaviour arises as a result of trying to deal with it. Repetitive and self-stimulating behaviours allow the child to cope with stress and avoid demanding situations. If they were adults, it is possible that they would turn to drugs.

This is why so many children with Down's syndrome also have autism. Their brains are easily damaged and they are very anxious people. Does testing for Down's syndrome during pregnancy with needling of the uterus cause stress to the foetus? These children used to be called 'delicate', which they are both mentally and physically, and are often not robust enough to deal with modern schooling and life, and the consequences are anxiety and autism.

There is no conventional treatment for autism other than avoidance of dietary intolerances, and speech and behavioural therapy. However, the Internet is full of histories of autistic children who have been considerably improved by homeopathy, including the 300 that the late Dr Smits treated. None of the official autism websites acknowledge this treatment. If you ask, they usually say that as it's not conventional medicine, it is not recommended, or that there is no research evidence to prove it is beneficial.

There is no way of testing children for metal toxicity, but they can be identified by assumption if the paediatrician is prepared to go down this path. The most likely metals in a child's system are mercury (from dentists and vaccines), and aluminium (vaccines) – both known to damage the brain. These substances can be chelated, that is, removed from the body and excreted in the stools and urine, by using homeopathy.

Damage from medication can be reversed by using the homeopathic remedy made from the same substance, e.g., penicillin 30C. Sugar should be avoided, but is often an addiction. This can be treated with saccharum 30C. There are remedies to detox anaesthetics, antibiotics, etc., and if the required remedy is not on the manufacturer's list, it can easily be made. This is called isotherapy – 'iso' meaning 'the same'; from the Greek 'isos' – 'equal'.

A common symptom of autism is fits. Children take conventional medication for fits, but homeopathic treatment can stop them without the need to keep taking medication.

People with autism also need supplementation with vitamins and micronutrients. They need at least vitamin C, zinc and magnesium, and omega-3 fish oils to restore brain function.

The treatment of children with homeopathy is complex and should be carried out by someone who is experienced.

There is a study being carried out in the USA to see if transfusion of umbilical-cord blood can help. Why bother with this potentially problematic method when homeopathy is cheap, effective, and available?

It may be that illness represents a disturbance in the fundamental energy system (vital force) of a person, and homeopathic remedies remind the body of its normal functioning so that it can be restored. Restoration will therefore occur at all levels.

Post-Traumatic Stress Disorder

This condition has been around since men have been fighting one another. In WW1 if you refused to fight due to fear you were shot for cowardice. PTSD has only recently had a name put to it and been recognised as a mental illness, but it was recognised in the homeopathic books dating from 1912, not by its modern name, but by recording accurately all the symptoms of the condition.

However, it is not only wars that cause it, and if you look you will find it everywhere. A young prison officer was on night duty. He was doing his rounds and checked on one prisoner and found him hanging and dead. He had a terrible shock and needed a year off work to recover.

All traffic incidents/accidents can cause it to some degree, usually depending on whether the result is minor or major. Shocks can also include hearing bad news, violence, being bullied, threatened, burgled, anything that causes severe, sudden fear, like watching someone being killed, including violent fantasy, whether online, on television programmes or films, and even in books.

The stress disorder lasts until the fear has been dealt with, as the brain puts the information in your subconscious (hard drive), from where the fear can escape at any time, and does so in flashbacks, episodes of anxiety or panic, and terrifying dreams.

Remedies for PTSD in homeopathy are found in the 'mind' section of the repertory, under the heading 'ailments from shock', as well as shock from fright, fear, and terror. It is also something that can be mentioned in relation to lots of other topics and issues, including dreams, accidents, amputations, bullying, danger, drowning, earthquakes, any significant previous events, fires, floods, being humiliated, killing, murder, pain, being pursued, rape, sexual perversity, attempted strangulation, being trapped, soldiers, spies, violence, graves/graveyards, war, and being wounded. From this list it is obvious that whatever symptoms a person with PTSD has, a homeopathic medicine can be found to help. The syndrome was known in Victorian times, as the symptoms are all in *Kent's Repertory*. Any person suffering from PTSD would benefit from homeopathy.

Psychopaths

It is possible that psychopaths could be viewed as having a chronic version of PTSD, in that they have often been subjected to repeated traumatic events during childhood, or even later in life, which have slowly rewired their brains (rather than a sudden shock), and turned them into the person that they become. I have never known this condition to have been treated in homeopathic practice, as psychopaths don't usually realise they are mentally ill, but it is theoretically possible.

But is homeopathy all in the mind? Why not use it more?

11

THE PLACEBO EFFECT

The word placebo derives from the Latin 'placere', meaning 'to please'. Recently, fewer new painkilling drugs have been getting through double-blind placebo-controlled trials – the gold standard for testing a drug's effectiveness. When researchers started looking closely at clinical trials of analgesics, in 1996 they found that an average of 27% of patients reported pain reduction from a new drug compared with a placebo. In 2013, it was 9%. What this showed was not that the drugs were less effective, but that the placebo response is growing bigger over time. And it is not just growing stronger in pain medicine. Placebos are also growing in strength in antidepressant and antipsychotic studies.

The placebo effect is very interesting. It is at the precise interface of mind and body, and is affected by everything from the drug adverts we see, to our interactions with doctors and nurses, as well as to the length of a clinical trial.

The science of placebos is bringing new understanding to why alternative treatments, like acupuncture and reiki, help some people. And it could also potentially allow us to one day prescribe smaller doses of pain drugs to help address the problem of people needing more and more analgesia for the same pain, which is an addiction.

There is no one placebo response. It's a family of overlapping psychological phenomena. Belief is the oldest medicine known to man.

The placebo effect is a surrogate marker for everything that surrounds a pill, and that includes rituals, symbols (like a stethoscope), doctor-patient encounters, and investigations. It is not just one thing. The family of placebo effects ranges from common sense to some difficult ideas. The simplest is the statistical phenomenon RTM, explained below.

Regression to the Mean (RTM)

When people first go to a doctor or start on a clinical trial, their symptoms might be particularly bad, but in the natural course of an illness symptoms may get better by themselves. In clinical studies of depression, researchers find that around one-third of patients get better without drugs or placebos. In other words, time itself is a kind of placebo effect that heals.

Sugar pills and active drugs can both change the way patients report symptoms.

Confirmation Bias

Patients believe they will get better when they are having treatment, so their focus changes. They pay closer attention to signs that they're getting better, and often ignore signs that they are getting worse. We also change our behaviour when we know we're being watched.

But the placebo effect is more than just bias…

Expectation and Learning

The placebo response is something we learn via cause and effect. When we take an active drug, we often feel better. This is a memory we revisit and recreate when taking a placebo. A study participant was hooked up to an electroshock machine. For each strong, painful shock, a red light was flashed on a screen the participant was looking at. For mild shocks, a green light was flashed. By the end of the experiment, when the participant saw the green light, they felt less pain, even when the shocks were at the highest setting.We get cues about how we should respond to pain – and medicines – from our environment. Studies show that post-operative patients whose painkillers are distributed by a hidden robot pump at an undisclosed time need twice as much of the drug to get the same pain-relieving effect as when the drug is injected by a nurse they could see. So awareness that you are being given something that is supposed to relieve pain seems to impact your perception of it working. Pain relief is stronger and more immediate when morphine is injected knowingly. Research also suggests that fake surgery – where doctors make some incisions but don't actually change anything – can be an even stronger placebo than pills. A 2014 systematic review of surgical placebos found that the fake surgeries led to improvements 75% of the time. In the case of surgery to relieve pain, one review found essentially no difference in outcomes between the real surgery and the fake ones.

There is also the nocebo effect, where negative expectations make people feel worse, especially when given bad news.

Pharmacological Conditioning

If you put patients on a drug to combat pain or deal with the symptoms of Parkinson's disease, then surreptitiously switch them over to a placebo, they still feel healing effects. When switched to placebos, a similar response in the brain occurs as with the real drug. Individual neurons in the brain of patients with Parkinson's disease will still respond to placebos as though they were actual anti-Parkinson's drugs, after such conditioning has taken place. This effect does not seem to last for long however, and as the patient has not actually had any medication, the underlying disease deteriorates, and when the effect of the placebo wears off, the patient may be worse than they would have been if they had had the active medication. The moral of this story is to never volunteer for a drug vs placebo trial.

The brain can learn to associate taking a pill with relief, and can produce the same brain chemicals when the drug is replaced with a placebo, if nutrition is good enough to manufacture the chemicals, and the brain is not depleting them too quickly. These results show that this is a neurobiological (a brain/body) phenomenon.

Social Learning

When study participants see another patient get relief from a placebo treatment, they have a greater placebo response – their mind probably thinks something like, *well, a friend says it works for them, so it should work for me...*

A Human Connection

Irritable bowel syndrome is a difficult condition to treat. People with IBS have to live with debilitating stomach cramps amongst other symptoms, and there are few effective treatments, and if doctors aren't sure of the underlying biological cause, they will not be able to treat it properly.

It is the type of ailment that can sometimes be derided as all in a patient's head, or a diagnosis of IBS can often be given prematurely when investigations fail to find the real cause of the symptoms. So, to see if usually intangible traits like warmth and empathy help make patients feel better, 260 participants were split into three groups. One group received sham acupuncture (meaning the needles were withdrawn before they touched the skin) from a practitioner who took extra time asking the patients about their life and struggles. He or she took pains to say things like, 'I can understand how difficult IBS must be for you'. A second group got sham acupuncture from a practitioner who did minimal talking. The third group was just put on a waiting list for treatment.

A caring provider can create a stronger placebo response than an apathetic one. The warm, friendly acupuncturist was able to produce better relief of symptoms. These results indicate that such factors as warmth, empathy, duration of interaction, and the communication of positive expectation might indeed significantly affect clinical outcome. Interviewers admitting students to medical schools should bear this in mind when selecting them. Medical students should also learn about the therapeutic consultation which is part of homeopathic training, so that they can use it in a positive way in the future.

The participants who received the augmented condition – the one in which the caregivers were extra attentive – reported better outcomes at the end of the three-week trial, compared with both the participants who received treatment as normal, and those waiting for treatment.

This may be the least understood component of placebos. It's not just about pills; it's about the environment a pill is taken in. It's about the person who gave it to you, and the rituals and encounters associated with them.

What Placebos Can and Cannot Do

Placebos seem to have the greatest power over symptoms that lie at the boundary between the physical and psychological.

A systematic review looked at 202 drug trials where a placebo group was compared to patients who received either a placebo or an active drug. It found that placebos seem to improve pain, nausea, asthma, and phobias, with more inconsistent results for outcomes like smoking, dementia, depression, obesity, hypertension, insomnia, and anxiety.

Placebos seem to alter our experience of symptoms, not their underlying causes. In an experiment, asthma patients were randomly sorted into four groups. One group received an inhaler with salbutamol, a drug that opens the airways. Another group was given an inhaler with a placebo. The third group had sham acupuncture. A fourth got nothing. The study authors evaluated lung function on two measurements: self-reporting from the patients on their asthma symptoms, and an objective measure of lung function.

From self-reporting of symptoms, the placebo, salbutamol, and sham acupuncture all seemed to be equally effective. The objective measure, however, showed only the salbutamol improved air flow. This does not mean that the self-reported improvements on the placebo didn't matter. In many illnesses patients would love a greater opportunity to ignore their symptoms. There are components in all the objectively measurable illnesses, like cancer and heart disease, and it is those symptoms that could be treated with placebos. Placebos influence the immune system via the psycho-neuro-hormono-immunology pathway.

Over the past 15 years, scientists have made some of their most interesting discoveries looking at how placebos have a powerful impact on the brain. Neuroscientists are beginning to uncover the underlying neural mechanisms that create the placebo response.

- Placebos can produce the release of opioids and other endorphins (chemicals that reduce pain) in the brain.
- Drugs that counteract the effects of opioids – such as naloxone – also counteract the placebo effect, which shows that placebos are indeed playing on the brain's natural pain-management circuitry.
- The periaqueductal grey matter, a region of the brain key for pain management, shows increased activity under placebos. Regions of the spinal cord that respond to pain show decreased activity under placebos, which suggests either the sensation of pain, or our perception of it, is diminished due to the placebos.
- Patients with dementia start to show a diminished placebo response. It is probably due to the degradation of their frontal lobes – the area of the brain that helps direct our subjective experience of the world.

346

Our understanding of all this is far from complete. Researchers still don't entirely understand how the brain processes pain. A lot of the brain regions implicated in the placebo response also play a role in emotions. So we don't yet know if placebos are actually reducing our sensation of pain, or just our interpretation of it.

There seems to be a placebo effect even if you tell patients that they are being given a placebo. Giving patients open-label placebos – sugar pills that the doctors admit *are* sugar pills – improved symptoms of certain chronic conditions that are among the hardest for doctors to treat, including irritable bowel syndrome and lower back pain.

There is a difference between belief and expectation, so while the patients may not believe the pill will work, they still unconsciously expect it to. This is because they still have a deep-seated conditioned memory for what it means to take a pill, as well as a conditioned memory for what it means to be in the care of another person. And these memories can indeed cause an expectation that can kick-start the analgesic effect in the brain. They don't have to be aware that it is happening.

Can Placebos be Integrated into Modern Medicine?

There is optimism that these discoveries can be used in clinical settings. There is still a lot of work left to do and certainly some of the findings are easier to implement than others. For instance, we should start with reminding doctors that they can help to relieve pain simply by being warm and caring to their patients. It may mean that patients are able to take less painkillers. This research only seems to have been carried out in the field of pain relief, and not in the curing of illness.

The main complaint thrown at homeopathy is that it is all a placebo. The healing power of the mind has become a key battleground in the fight against irrational thinking (the science of medicine). The art of medicine should be that all patients are individuals with their own personal past history, set of genes, and pattern of expression of illnesses.

How can modern medicine be rational when it is governed by profit for big pharma? In over 30 years in GP I accumulated a number of bribes from drug reps: small things like bookmarks, which all had the name of the manufacturer and the medication easily visible to remind you to prescribe them. In fact, none of them is in use today. Why not, if they were as wonderful as the reps made out?

Animals

It is difficult to study the placebo response in animals, but it is well known that animals also react positively to human kindness. Homeopathy works well in animals as well.

A farmer was having considerable trouble with mastitis in his milking cows. It was running at 25%. He asked a homeopathic vet to treat them. Antibiotics for mastitis are expensive and time-consuming, in that they have to be administered via the teat by the cowman, and the milk has to be thrown away.

The vet asked the farmer if he would allow him to do a small trial. The farmer agreed and the vet gave the cowman two bottles marked 'A' and 'B'. He was asked to empty one of the bottles into the first drinking trough, and the other bottle into the second trough. There were two groups of cows that each went into the same stalls to be milked, and always drank from the same troughs. After two weeks the vet and the cowman assessed the level of mastitis, and found that in one group it had reduced to 2% and in the other group had stayed the same. They then changed the water and carried out the same process, but emptied the bottles 'A' and 'B' into the opposite troughs. Two weeks later they reassessed. The other group of cows had reduced mastitis levels, and the first group had gone up by a few per cent, but not to previous levels, showing that the treatment had had a lasting effect. They then broke the code to find that the 25% group had received the placebo, and the 2% group had received the active treatment. The farmer continued to treat all his cows with the homeopathic remedies, and had no major problems with mastitis subsequently.

Clinical trials in homeopathy are notoriously difficult to do. It is not possible to test one disease versus one drug as it is in conventional medicine, as each patient is taken as an individual with their own pattern of past history and current variable symptoms. Consequently, even patients with the same problem will need different remedies. Homeopathy is the only discipline that takes the patient's individual mental symptoms, beliefs, and working of the mind into account. The doctor keeps an open mind and listens to the patient tell their own story and explanations of feelings. You should ask them: 'What does this feel like?'; 'Tell me more about the pain.' Or, 'Explain this or that feeling...' Using this method, you can find out what really makes a patient ill, that is, how they respond to their problem or stress.

Patients frequently say that despite having seen many doctors in the past, nobody has ever asked these sorts of questions. At the end of a homeopathic-based consultation, which may be therapeutic in its own right, and therefore having a strong placebo effect, the patient may be asked if they feel they need any medication. They might think they have enough insight into their situation to proceed without any.

If you are lucky, the placebo effect makes you better because it has rewired your brain temporarily, because usually the placebo effect wears off quite quickly. When homeopathy cures, however, it seems to rewire the brain permanently.

It is a pity that if the scientific world feels that the placebo effect is so noticeable in homeopathy, then why is it not noticeable in conventional medicine? I never saw anyone who was cured of any chronic disease with conventional medicine, even taking the placebo effect into account. Conventional medicine does not tackle the emotional component of disease, which is what homeopathy is good at.

The proponents of conventional, Western medicine are rational, reductionist, and rooted in the material world. They think of the body as a machine and usually thoughts, beliefs and emotions don't feature in treatment for their patients' medical conditions.

Doctors use physical methods like blood tests, scans, drugs, and surgery to diagnose and fix the damaged part of patients. In real life, parts are not damaged, but are subject to chemical change, electromagnetic change, and psycho-neuro-hormono-immunology. In other words, a cascade of interdependent changes.

The objectors may think of homeopathy as being absurd, but if they had been sitting in my chair for 30 years, and saw what damage drugs do and how they never cure, they would be pleased to be able to prescribe homeopathic remedies. Patients have more sense than they are often given credit for, and mostly choose to try homeopathy. I can only hope that writers of books and websites against homeopathy never find themselves in a position where they have to go along the conventional medical route with a serious disease, or have to take medicines which affect them negatively. At least homeopathy does no harm.

If a placebo is so important as a criticism of homeopathy, why does no one teach doctors to make positive use of it?

Think how much money the NHS would be able to save if a proportion of patients were treated with placebos. The answer, of course, is to do with funding. The problem is that doctors think that treating patients with placebo tablets is illegal, immoral, and have no idea how to handle it. Big pharma would not be supportive, as it would receive no financial gain.

Most of the time, doctors in general practice, particularly as patients now rarely see the same doctor twice, have no idea what the outcome of their interactions with the patients has been. In homeopathic practice, to get our postgraduate revalidation, everyone had to keep an outcome score for each patient that they saw. The outcome score is a standardised score in homeopathy that follows the path of the patient's recovery.

A paper, written in 2005, studied 6,544 patients who attended Bristol Homeopathic Hospital outpatients department with a wide range of conditions. They had all been everywhere and seen everybody, and homeopathy was a last resort for them. Everyone had the outcome score assessed for the results of the treatment, and on average there was a 70% improvement. Given that patients were using homeopathy as a last resort, this was an amazing improvement in their health. If this were repeated throughout the NHS, think what it would mean in terms of health improvement. Demand for services would go down because people would feel better, and would not need to see a doctor so frequently. The patients seen at the Bristol Homeopathic Hospital had dermatological, urological, gynaecological, rheumatological, gastroenterological, oncological, otolaryngological, cardiological, respiratory, and psychiatric conditions and diseases. The NHS would not be in such a dire financial situation if all doctors were trained in homeopathy.

Unfortunately, the hospital was recently closed down, despite its outstandingly good results, as the managers felt that keeping it open was a waste of money that could be used for other services.

Using the same method, I kept my own personal outcome scores for my patients, and found the same pattern as they did in Bristol. In fact, one of the medical students came and assessed the outcomes, particularly patients who did not return for a follow-up appointment. She found that they did not return mainly because they were much improved and satisfied with their progress.

There have been a number of notable epidemics that have been stopped using homeopathic medicine. In 1971 in São Paulo, Brazil, there was a severe outbreak of meningitis in the city. There were over 30,000 cases and services were overwhelmed. It was due to type B meningococcus. At that time there were no conventional vaccines available, so the public health system decided to use the homeopathic meningococcus vaccine. The Department of Public Health, who did not believe that the medication would work, divided the city into two halves, and gave one half the meningococcus in a homeopathic potency, and the other half nothing. The trial had to be stopped after a short while because the incidence of meningitis in the treated part of the city dropped dramatically. Then the whole city was given the meningococcus remedy and the epidemic disappeared.

More recently, an outbreak of Weil's disease, spread by rats in the rainy season in Cuba, was treated with the homeopathic vaccine. Weil's disease occurred in Cuba annually, and was very difficult to treat and eradicate. There is no conventional vaccine or treatment for it. After the homeopathic vaccine was introduced the epidemics disappeared. It would seem that this method of medicine should be looked into further, and not dismissed out of hand.

12

HOMEOPATHY

The main problem with the homeopathic method is that detractors and sceptics think that it's implausible that something as dilute as the remedies appear to be cannot possibly work. This is nothing new. The Faculty of Homeopathy was founded in 1844 in London, to try to cope with this problem. It was well before the Royal College of Physicians was established.

Dr James Compton Burnett (1840–1901) was a pioneer in his work as a homeopathic physician. He wrote a factual account of his conversion to homeopathy in his book, *Fifty Reasons for Being a Homeopath*. He looked after a ward in a London hospital, admitting children who were very ill with fevers, which were common in Victorian London. It must have been a terrible job, because most of the children died quite rapidly, and part of his days involved writing many death certificates.

One evening, feeling very dispirited, he went out for a meal with a friend who was a homeopathic doctor. His friend noticed how gloomy he looked as he told his story, then asked if he had thought of homeopathy for the children. Burnett lost his temper and said: 'This isn't a joke. Children are dying and I am thinking of giving it all up and being a farmer.' He said he was tired of being unable to help the children and felt powerless when they died. He felt he was not doing any good for his patients.

His friend asked him again if he had considered using homeopathic medicines, and he replied that he had been taught at Cambridge that homeopathy was a farce, even a disgrace, and orthodox doctors were forbidden to use it. Sound familiar? His friend stated his case and suggested a book he might read, and if it struck him that the author was a charlatan, then he should throw the book and the ideas away. But if he found that the book had real substance, then try it. What was there to lose?

On his way home he purchased the book, but felt as if he were about to commit a crime. Then he thought of the high mortality of the cases on the ward. He read the book and decided that either the author was a fool, or there was real merit in his ideas.

He felt cheered up for a while, then scepticism crept in. If the book were true, why had this method not already been implemented? He decided to try it at the bedside, and prove once and for all that it did not work and was a sham.

He looked up the remedy to give to children with a fever and decided to get some aconite, which was given to the children by a nurse as soon as they were admitted to the ward, but only to half of them, to see what happened. He was certain that the remedy would make no difference.

The next day he was keen to find out what had happened, and on entering the ward was nonplussed to find that the children treated with aconite had been cured of their fevers, and were well enough to be playing and ready for discharge. One child, however, had come out in a measles rash, and the untreated children were the same – or worse.

He asked the nurse to continue with the aconite, and day after day, the results were the same, until she refused to not give it to every child, and so many lives were saved.

Burnett learnt from this experience, took up homeopathy, and built up a satisfying, busy private practice. That was 150 years ago.

Dr Luc Montagnier, the French virologist, surprised the scientific community by his strong support for homeopathy, despite winning the Nobel Prize in Physiology or Medicine in 2008, of which one half was awarded jointly to Montagnier and Françoise Barré-Sinoussi for their discovery of the human immunodeficiency virus (HIV), and the other half to Harald zur Hausen for his discovery of human papilloma viruses causing cervical cancer.

In an interview published in *Science* magazine, Professor Montagnier expressed support for the often maligned and misunderstood medical speciality of homeopathic medicine. Although homeopathy has been used for over 200 years all over the world, and is the leading alternative treatment used in South America, the USA and Europe, conventional physicians express scepticism about its efficacy because of its small doses.

Most clinical research conducted on homeopathic medicines that has been published in peer-review journals has shown positive clinical results, especially in the treatment of respiratory allergies, influenza, fibromyalgia, rheumatoid arthritis, childhood diarrhoea, post-surgical abdominal surgery recovery, attention deficit disorder, and reduction in the side effects of conventional cancer treatments. In addition to clinical trials, several hundred basic scientific studies have confirmed the biological activity of homeopathic medicines.

As well as the wide variety of basic scientific evidence and clinical research, further evidence for homeopathy is based on the fact that it gained widespread popularity in the USA and Europe during the nineteenth century due to the impressive results people experienced in the treatment of epidemics, including cholera, typhoid, yellow fever, scarlet fever, and influenza. Montagnier, who is also founder and president of the World Foundation for AIDS Research and Prevention, said that he could not say that homeopathy is right in everything, but what he could say is that the high dilutions (used in homeopathy) are right. High dilutions of something are not nothing. They are water structures which mimic the original molecules.

Here, Montagnier is making reference to his experimental research that confirms one of the controversial features of homeopathic medicine, which uses doses of substances that undergo sequential dilution with vigorous shaking in-between each dilution. Although it is common for modern-day scientists to assume that none of the original molecules remain in solution, Montagnier's research (and that of many of his colleagues) has verified that electromagnetic signals of the original medicine remain in the water and have definite biological effects. Homeopathic medicines work by physics and not by chemistry as conventional medicines do.

Montagnier recently moved to a new position at Shanghai University in China, often referred to as 'China's MIT' (Massachusetts Institute of Technology), where he works in an institute bearing his name. His work focuses on a new scientific movement at the crossroads of physics, biology, and medicine: the phenomenon of electromagnetic waves produced by

DNA in water. He and his team study both the theoretical basis and the possible applications.

He affirms that these new observations will lead to novel treatments for many common chronic diseases and disorders, including – but not limited to – autism, Alzheimer's, and Parkinson's disease.

French retirement laws do not allow Montagnier, who is past retirement age, to work at a public institute, thereby limiting access to research funding. He acknowledges that getting research funds from big pharma and other conventional research-funding agencies is unlikely due to the atmosphere of antagonism to homeopathy.

In addition to Montagnier and the research of the late Jacques Benveniste, a biologist and immunologist, is the weighty opinion of Brian Josephson, PhD, who, like Montagnier, is a Nobel-Prize-winning scientist. He responded to an article on homeopathy:

Regarding your comments on claims made for homeopathy: criticisms centred around the vanishingly small number of solute molecules present in a solution after it has been repeatedly diluted are beside the point, since advocates of homeopathic remedies attribute their effects not to molecules present in the water, but to changes in the structure of the water.

Simple-minded analysis may suggest that water, being a fluid, cannot have a structure of the kind that such a picture would demand. But cases such as that of liquid crystals, which while flowing like an ordinary fluid can maintain an ordered structure over macroscopic distances, show the limitations of such ways of thinking. There have not, to the best of my knowledge, been any refutations of homeopathy that remain valid after this particular point is taken into account.

A related topic is the phenomenon – claimed by the late Jacques Benveniste's colleague Yolène Thomas (and by others) to be well-established experimentally – known as 'memory of water'. If valid, this would be of greater significance than homeopathy itself, and it attests to the limited vision of the modern scientific community that, far from testing such claims, the only response has been to dismiss them out of hand. Josephson, who is an emeritus professor of Cambridge University, was asked by *New Scientist* editors how he became an advocate of unconventional ideas. He responded:

> *I went to a conference where the French immunologist Jacques Benveniste was talking for the first time about his discovery that water has a 'memory' of compounds that were once dissolved in it – which might explain how homeopathy works. His findings provoked irrationally strong reactions from scientists, and I was struck by how badly he was treated.*

Josephson went on to describe how many scientists today suffer from 'pathological disbelief' – that is, they maintain an unscientific attitude that is embodied by the statement, 'even if it were true I would not believe it'.

Montagnier concluded the interview for *Science* magazine when asked if he were concerned that he was drifting into pseudoscience, and he replied adamantly: 'No, because it's not pseudoscience. It's not quackery. These are real phenomena which deserve further study.'

What is Homeopathy?

Samuel Hahnemann was born in 1755 in Meissen, Saxony (now officially the Free State of Saxony), in east-central Germany. He qualified as a conventional doctor and went to work in a mining town in the Harz Mountains. The miners and their families were always ill with problems that he could do nothing about. He recognised their poverty and poor diets, and the miners' lung conditions, but the treatments at that time consisted of things like leeching, purging, and poisonous medicines, none of which worked and made him feel helpless. He thought he could no longer work as a doctor. As he was very good at languages, he moved to Leipzig and worked translating medical literature. He was asked to translate Cullen's *Materia Medica*.

In 1755 Cullen was the professor of chemistry at the University of Edinburgh, and in 1760 he began lecturing in Materia Medica as well. He'd written a book describing every plant that was used in medicine. It was therefore a textbook of herbal medicines. Hahnemann knew a lot about plants, and that they could be poisonous as well as helping heal in a slow manner. When he read the description of the way in which the medicine cinchona,

Peruvian bark, was said to work to heal malaria, he thought Cullen was wrong.

He decided to test it on himself, so obtained some powdered bark, and took some each day. He recorded everything that happened to him. After a few doses he began to feel unwell, but continued. He soon felt so unwell that he had to stop taking it. When he recovered, he looked at what he had written, and realised that all the symptoms he had experienced from the mild poisoning were the same as if he had actually had malaria. He went to the extensive library in Dresden to read the history of medicine books to see if this was a known phenomenon. He discovered that ancient Greek doctors had used the 'like treats like' effect, but when their influence disappeared, so did the method. He realised he had discovered a method that could be developed to effectively treat people.

Hahnemann spent the rest of his life discovering new medicines and pursuing the systematic investigation of how to treat using this method. In 1796, he published his first paper on this type of treatment, for which he coined the German word 'homöopathie' – combining the Greek 'homoios', meaning 'like', with 'patheia', meaning 'feeling'. He taught how to look for all the symptoms that the patient describes, and match them with the poisoning symptoms of the remedy.

There were many epidemics, especially in children, and one of the first remedies he studied was belladonna. He knew that the poisonous symptoms of the plant atropa belladonna were the same as the symptoms that the children who were developing scarlet fever showed, so he offered it to the families in which there was scarlet fever. He also gave it as a prevention to the unaffected children.

He soon realised that although the children were cured, they often had an aggravation of their symptoms first. He was collecting the plants himself, soaking them in alcohol and water to leach out the essence, and then giving drops of it to the children. As some of the children became worse, he felt that the dose was obviously too strong, so he started mixing one drop of the solution with 99 drops of a water/alcohol mixture. The alcohol was there as a preservative. He labelled the doses as '1C' (one in a hundred – the 'centesimal' scale of potency). He felt it was not enough to just mix the plant and water drops together and dilute them. He wanted to activate the medicine, so he succussed it (shook vigorously) by stoppering the bottle, then striking it against a book. This preparation was then tested on the patients and found to work, and gave fewer aggravations. A 2C preparation was then made, with one drop from the 1C solution, and 99 drops of the water with alcohol, before being tested on the children. Continuing in this manner, he found that the best preparation for curing without aggravations was a 6C mix.

Throughout Hahnemann's life he looked for new remedies – from plants, animal poisons like bee stings, and poisonous medicines like arsenic and mercury, which, at the time, were used to treat syphilis, but they poisoned the patients rather than cured the disease. He treated Napoléon's army when they were camped outside Leipzig and had epidemics of cholera and typhus. When he became successful, the doctors and pharmacists ran him out of town because he cured more patients than they did, so his family was often moving house. After his wife died he moved to Paris, and had an extremely successful practice.

People came from all over the world to see Hahnemann, and he trained many doctors, who took the methods they'd learnt back to their own countries, which is how they arrived in London and were taken up by British royalty. If Queen Victoria's doctors had allowed her to call for her homeopathic physician when Albert was dying, history might have been quite different.

Homeopathy has moved on in the last 200 years. It is now popular in most countries, but conventional medicine still has problems with it. Many new medicines have had to be made to suit modern diseases, and often to deal with the side effects of modern medicines, like antibiotics and chemotherapy.

New methods of producing the remedies include different scales. Decimal ('D') is one drop in nine drops of water and alcohol. 'M' denotes one drop in 1,000, and 'LM' denotes one drop in 50,000. These other potencies are more often given in chronic diseases that have been present for a long time.

There is no disease that homeopaths have not been asked to treat. Often disease is complicated by effects from drugs, and needs to be treated in layers. You really only *truly* heal someone if you cure their inner self, as symptoms are only the external manifestation of what is going on deep inside. If doctors really want to cure or heal, they must learn homeopathy. This way you never have a damaged patient. All the complaints departments could be closed. Think of the money that would save.

There are homeopathic vaccines which have no side effects, and prevent flu and all the childhood diseases. They are called nosodes. I often use the herpes simplex nosode for people with recurrent cold sores. I think the stopping of severe, recurrent cold sores has impressed more patients than other conditions. The herpes zoster nosode treats the after-effects of shingles and any other nosode relevant to the 'never well since' syndrome, like glandular fever. There are plenty of treatments for viral infections, whereas there are none in conventional medicine.

Homeopathic remedies are always safe, as they either work, that is, the remedy is correct, or they don't work, which means the wrong remedy has been chosen. It is as if the origins of the disease have been targeted by the medicine, and any damage has been repaired and switched into normal operating mode. At follow-up consultations, you ask about not only whether symptoms have improved, but if the patient feels generally better in themself. The use of homeopathic medicines would revolutionise the treatment of mental health problems.

The sceptics seem to think that there is no evidence for the effectiveness of homeopathy. They just need to read the right journals. The *British Journal of Homoeopathy* (BJH) was published from 1884 and became the *British Homoeopathic Journal* (BHJ) in 1911. It obtained its current name *Homeopathy* in 2001. The *British Medical Journal* (BMJ) was founded in 1840. Doctors do not claim that homeopathy works; we see it every day. We do see private patients, but charge them considerably less than conventional specialists do. The remedies are not a misuse of resources, and time spent with a patient is never a misuse.

The medicines are stored in small glass bottles and not in blister packs, which is much more environmentally friendly. The manufacture of the medicines only needs the smallest amount of the raw material to make many doses, which is also much more environmentally friendly. There are no side effects, which is patient-friendly, and the patient is never at risk from the medicines or from a misdiagnosis. In fact, I have often been able to put a name to what the patient has wrong by just listening to them properly.

Patients come for homeopathic treatment when they feel let down by standard treatment. The patient may or may not come with an official diagnosis by the NHS system. As doctors we know what the diagnosis means. Non-medically qualified homeopaths without much experience may have difficulty interpreting a diagnosis. There are no non-medically qualified members of the Faculty of Homeopathy, and we have not chosen this route because of the ability to earn a lot of money, but because we have seen the help that homeopathy can be.

Why do sceptics think that homeopathic vaccines are a con, when they have never looked at the evidence, and never had to sit in the doctor's chair and listen to mothers' worries about symptoms after a child's first vaccine? Patients may lie, or tell a version of the truth about things like stopping smoking, but not if their child is involved. I can only hope that the sceptics are never struck down by a disease that modern medicine can do little about, and never have to go abroad to a country where they are advised to have a number of vaccines, or come up against a disease for which there are no vaccines, like MRSA.

The Faculty of Homeopathy in London governs the practice of doctors, vets, dentists, and other registered practitioners. The Faculty keeps a list on its website of everyone registered. There is three-year training involved in learning homeopathy, with the MFHom exam at the end. Members can be elected as fellows. All registered practitioners have to keep up their postgraduate education.

Non-medically qualified practitioners can also be found online. They have qualifications from schools of homeopathy in the UK.

Herbal Medicines

Do not confuse homeopathy with herbal medicines. The system of treating people with herbs is a very old practice, and involves picking the plants and either infusing them in alcohol, or drying the plants and making tablets out of them. The tablets have to be swallowed in the same way as conventional medication and are absorbed from the bowel, unlike homeopathic medicines which are absorbed from the mouth and go straight to the brain.

Herbal remedies might help some problems, but if stopped, the symptoms of a chronic disease may return, as with conventional medication. If the medication is stopped the problem may return. Herbal medicines act via chemistry, as do drugs, but homeopathic medicines work by physics, getting to the cause of the illness and therefore the cure.

Money

The NHS is in difficulty because it cannot fund all the treatment that so many sick people need. Drug companies have to fund research for their next drug and pass the costs on to the NHS. The medication you can buy over the counter helps to fund research, but most of it is only available OTC now because it is not very effective.

Homeopathic remedies are cheap, and can be easily and quickly made. If there were a serious pandemic of flu again, a homeopathic vaccine would be available virtually immediately, made from the actual virus responsible. Conventional medicine cannot do this, as its method of preparing the relevant vaccine takes months, especially in the numbers that would be needed. Coronavirus (COVID-19) is a respiratory virus, and in India, those who have taken homeopathic medicines have had a lower death rate. At the time of writing, the demand for homeopathic remedies has increased during the ongoing coronavirus pandemic, not just in India, but all over the world.

How to Use Homeopathic Medicines

Homeopathic remedies have the advantage of being able to be prepared in various forms: drops (liquid), sugar pills, lactose tablets, powder, or tiny granules. They can be used at any age, given to any animal, and even used if the patient is unconscious. They never harm an unborn baby. All are absorbed from the mouth and are never swallowed (tablets, for example, can be sucked), so consequently never upset the stomach. A drop of arnica under the tongue of unconscious people who have been injured would get them better quicker and out of intensive care sooner, thus saving money. The dose is the same for a baby or a tall man, for a bird or an elephant.

It is easy to have a few remedies in the house like arnica 6C for injuries. It is also easy to buy remedies online. They are cheap and never wear out like modern drugs, which have a shelf life. Manufacturers have to obey the law and put a use-by date on the label, but a colleague of mine was asked by the wife of a doctor who had just died to take his homeopathic remedies away for her. He did so, and realised that some of them were over 40 years old. He used them in his practice and they still worked.

Learning homeopathy changed my life in practice. I asked my partners if they would be happy for me to use it in the surgery and they were divided. Two thought it was rubbish and I would soon find out that it wasn't worth the effort. I wonder if they realised that all the antibiotics they prescribed may have altered biomes and caused many problems later. Two supported me and two were ambivalent, saying that as long as it caused no difficulties I could go ahead. There was only ever one complaint, from the senior partner, that he had been called out at 9.00 p.m.

one night to see a child whom I had seen that evening, i.e., three hours before, with earache, and the homeopathic remedies hadn't worked yet. He suggested I always treat ear infections with antibiotics, but even if I had, there would have been no improvement, as it takes longer than three hours for them to start working.

Once word got around that I was using homeopathy, people started coming to see me specially for treatment, as their problems had not been solved by the other doctors. I still meet people in the town who remember being helped considerably by the treatment. I converted one partner by curing his son, a keen cricketer, of hay fever. I also had medicines to treat children with croup. The receptionist would let me know that one had arrived, and I would prepare a glass of water and a tablet of aconite and one of spongia, which I kept in my drawer. I would dissolve the tablets and ask the mum to give a dose every few minutes. Usually after about half an hour the attack was over. I never needed to refer a child for admission using this method.

I frequently saw my partners' patients who came for homeopathic treatment because the conventional had not worked. I always discussed the method with patients and was only ever refused twice – once by a lady who said that her husband would not allow her to take it, and once by a lady who said I must be mad if I thought she would take it. I also treated a patient's flock of budgerigars with aconite in their drinking water, and a vet's dog that had been shot with arnica. The vet took an interest in homeopathy after that incident.

I used homeopathic remedies every day and they never let me down. After some years I had quite a lot of experience and decided to write a thesis for fellowship. Around that time I met a young man with haemophilia. His mum brought him to see me in desperation. She had just been told he had hepatitis and HIV antibodies and there was no treatment. Could I help? The treatment I gave him, then his brother, then three more boys, stalled their antibodies and made a huge difference to their lives. They all became fitter, had fewer infections, and needed less factor VIII to stop bleeds. Because they had fewer bleeds it cost the NHS considerably less. One adult had just been in hospital with his first episode of AIDS. Pneumocystis pneumonia had left him feeling very unwell. He had been discharged with a cough, wheeze, loss of appetite, night sweats, loss of weight, and an uncertain future. He was taking antibiotics long-term, but they did not seem to be resolving his problem. After calcium carbonate 200C, however, his pneumonia cleared up in days. All the patients with haemophilia I treated improved, but the consultant told everyone that anybody who had homeopathic treatment would not be able to be treated for haemophilia by him, and would have to go elsewhere. I was consequently not able to follow patients up long-term.

Since then I have read three papers about haemophilia (one Spanish, one Russian, and one Indian), which showed exactly the same as I had found. The Indian study found that homeopathy provided better pain relief, reduced the frequency and severity of bleeding, improved mental well-being and behaviour, reduced absenteeism from school and work, and reduced the need for costly clotting factor concentrates. All patients' general health improved and they needed considerably less factor VIII. Everyone with hepatitis and HIV antibodies did much better than expected. If this had been reproduced in the UK, it would have saved the NHS a lot of money. I sent the thesis I'd written to The Haemophilia Society charity, but they ignored it.

I also wrote a paper about endometriosis, and worked out that it was caused by retrograde menstrual blood (which is normal) not being absorbed by the peritoneum as usual, because the immune system had been damaged, usually by antibiotics, causing a damaged biome. There has been a serious increase in the number of women with endometriosis, and it causes infertility and menstrual problems. It is difficult to treat with conventional medication, and the first lady I encountered came to see me because she wanted to become pregnant and when endometriosis was discovered the treatment she was offered was the pill. As she was in her mid-thirties she did not want to take it. Happily, homeopathy solved both problems.

The article I subsequently wrote about endometriosis for *Health and Homeopathy*, the magazine of the British Homeopathic Association, was published online and I have had emails and phone calls from all over the UK and many foreign countries about this illness. I usually suggest that people print the article out and take it with them to see a homeopath near them.

I also treated three patients with post-polio syndrome. They had all had polio when young and eventually suffered with leg pains that hampered any ability to walk. One lady was so impressed with the results of the treatment that she wrote an article for the *Birmingham Mail*, then allowed me to use it for an article in the *Health and Homeopathy* magazine. I still get phone calls about this article as well, because it offers some help when the NHS offers none. I prescribed the polio nosode and other remedies according to the patient's reactions and symptoms.

It would appear that homeopathy offers treatment when none is otherwise offered, especially where there is chronic disease or multiple pathology, particularly mental health problems. There are rarely complaints about treatment, and I was Chairman of the Disciplinary & Professional Performance Committee for the Faculty of Homeopathy for some years, so would have known if there were. There was very little to attend to.

Patients were happy to try homeopathic remedies and usually did well on them. They remember the occasions still, and remind me about them when I see them.

Homeopathy is good at treating anxiety, depression, and other mental health problems – an area where little is available to help.

Although there is a lot of learning to do to become experienced with homeopathy, as the NHS is divided into such narrow disciplines, it would not be too difficult to introduce remedies, especially for acute medicine and paediatrics. The difficulty lies in chronic disease, especially the emotional problems associated with it. To me the training in homeopathy gave me the ability to treat people who would have never got better without it.

If homeopathy is so successful when other methods have failed, costs very little compared with the usual treatments, if there even are any, and causes no side effects or damage, it seems a shame not to take advantage of it. Patients would benefit, and the NHS finances would benefit. The only losers would be big pharma, as less of their medications would be used.

The trouble is that the NHS and the people who run it (doctors, nurses and administrators, etc.) have the system set up the way they need it for modern surgery, diagnoses and treatment. The change would be that homeopathy can be slowly and gradually introduced into each department. Homeopathy can never replace the surgery needed for many situations, as often disease, when discovered, may need radical treatment. It could never replace stents and bypasses for coronary heart disease, nor surgery for cancer that is advanced. However, it can be given alongside these treatments, and when given alongside chemotherapy does not stop it working, but helps with the problem of side effects.

There will always be patients who are too ill to recover, but the vast majority are not, and would be glad of some extra help with their problems. It is an ideal method for general practice, and pharmacists would find the remedies easy to source, as there are many manufacturers in the UK. The remedies also take up little space; I kept over 200 different ones in three drawers of my desk, and would often give the patient one tablet at the time, and two more to take home. Think of how much homeopathy could help with antibiotic resistance, which is increasingly becoming a problem.

Homeopathy is also planet-friendly, as only plants, minerals, venoms, bacteria, viruses (taken from swabs of a patient with the disease), and animal secretions are used, and there is no harm done in the process.

13

HOW TO RELIEVE ANXIETY
AND BUILD COPING SKILLS

The first thing to learn is to recognise your own symptoms of anxiety. This means being aware of what is happening to your body. Look at yourself in the mirror. What is your posture like? Are you often clenching your teeth, frowning, screwing up your eyes, talking too much, or too little, fiddling with your hair, scratching or rubbing your skin, picking your fingernails, biting your nails, or fidgeting too much, like sitting with your knees crossed but continuously moving your feet? Are you ever still?

It is your habits that cause most problems. It would be wise to look at them with mindfulness, and see what can be changed or modified. Any behaviour, including posture, should be checked. This especially relates to the symptoms of obsessive-compulsive states. If you have good insight into what is going on in your mind and body, you can try to modify it yourself, or get some help.

You need to learn to sit and stand in a good posture, like the mountain posture in yoga, or the military posture, with hands by your side, as actors do, or clasped lightly in your lap. When you sit down choose a chair that will support your back. Slouching on the sofa is bad posture and can lead to back and neck pain. If you sit at a desk for a long period you will naturally slouch. Take regular breaks to stand up and stretch. Imagine being pulled upwards by a string attached to the top of your head. This will help align your body and stretch your spine. Never hold your phone between your ear and shoulder as it strains your neck, and upper back and shoulders. Never thrust your chin forward, which is done subconsciously, and can be a symptom of aggression. Body alignment in yoga poses provides feedback to the parasympathetic nervous system via the vagus nerve, and tones it up to work more efficiently.

Look at your workstation and see what effect it is having on your posture and muscle tension. Even washing-up and other housework can have an effect on the upper body, because sinks may not be at the right height for the person using them, and household equipment may need effort to use, so muscles are strained. Always stand with your feet apart, with toes facing forward for balance. A good posture reflects confidence. Looking at the ground a lot indicates low mood, so practise looking upwards and around.

Muscles can be painful if they are overused in the wrong anatomical position. If you are having muscular problems due to stress, take advice from an osteopath, or seek advice at your local gym for exercises to do to strengthen these muscles. The eventual effects of tense muscles can result in fibromyalgia syndrome in younger people, and polymyalgia rheumatica in older.

If you cannot sort your own posture out, get some advice from a practitioner trained in the Alexander technique, or take-up an activity like yoga or dancing. Once you realise what anxiety is doing to you, then you may be able to calm things down.

Anxiety shows itself in many other ways. It is important if you are addicted to something to realise that the underlying problem is probably anxiety. If you can accept that and put strategies into place, things should improve.

The late Dr Claire Weekes MBE, who was an Australian GP and physician, said in her book, *Self Help for Your Nerves*, that the most important thing in getting better is first of all to face up to the problem; then get a proper diagnosis and understand that the physical effects are all secondary to anxiety. Truly accept that your symptoms are due to anxiety and not because of something else, which

387

your imagination might sometimes try to tell you. This usually means that when your symptoms arise, reassure yourself that you know what is causing them and what they are, and then you won't be as frightened by them. Thinking that it's only your nerves can help to calm you down. Then 'float' through them, which means deep breathing and relaxation, even if you have an attack in a supermarket, for example. Do not be afraid of your symptoms. They can feel frightening, but are only due to overactivity of your nerves.

If you suffer from anxiety attacks buy a small bottle of aconite 30C. Take it with you wherever you go, and suck repeatedly if an attack occurs. My patients have usually found this very helpful. You are not supposed to run away when an attack strikes, but have to breathe slowly and calmly. If you then let time pass, things will improve considerably, because you are training your brain.

Breathing with the stomach is the key to relaxation. When you are tense your stomach muscles are also tense and you breathe with your upper chest. As this is shallow breathing, you may hyperventilate in order to get more air into your lungs. This will make you feel dizzy and faint.

Everyone should develop strategies to nurture their mental health, like eating a healthy diet, yoga or exercise classes, breathing exercises, looking into philosophical thoughts and sayings, singing, music, poetry, or prayer. In this situation, religion is said to be 'the opium of the people', as the German philosopher Karl Marx said.

Sleep

The pineal gland at the base of your brain controls the diurnal variation in your body. This means it tells you when you are ready for bed, and wakes you up. It is therefore very important to keep this gland working properly, and to do so it needs constant rewiring. Consequently, sleep is extremely important for mental health. You should go to bed at the same time every day and also get up at the same time.

Sleeping for at least eight hours as an adult protects you from heart attacks and strokes. People who sleep fewer than six hours a night produce more of the hunger hormone ghrelin, and less of the hormone leptin, which makes you feel full. As a consequence they eat approximately 300 calories more each day, and so may put on weight. They also get colds more often and are more vulnerable to cancer.

Dreams transfer memories from short-term to long-term storage, and strip away the memories' original emotional components. However, if your mental health is already disturbed, it will have an effect on your sleep patterns. Children who want to sleep with the light on because they are scared of the dark, are often specifically afraid of things like zombies! It's very difficult to persuade them that zombies are a figment of an adult's imagination and not fact.

If you are unable to get off to sleep, it is usually because you are anxious and your thoughts go around and around in your mind, and will not settle down. Try the five B's...

The Five B's for Relaxation

1. BED: Lie in bed in a comfortable position in which to relax. Practise this method in bed if you cannot get off to sleep, or if you have waken too early.

2. BREATHING: Lie with your hands on your lower stomach and breathe through your nose. Let your hands

move up and down as you breathe with your stomach. Do not breathe with your chest, as this is tense, anxious breathing, but breathing with your abdomen is relaxing. Inhale for a count of two and breathe out for a count of five. As you breathe out slowly your pulse rate drops, your adrenaline levels fall, and you begin to relax. As you breathe in, think of the word 'peace'. As you breathe out, think of the word 'calm'.

3. BODY: Now relax your whole body, bit by bit, starting with the feet and working upwards. Imagine your feet feel like lumps of lead and they're sinking into the bed. Make your way up the whole body, naming the parts as you go, not forgetting the pelvic floor. If any part will not relax, tense it up first.

4. BRAIN: This is the most important organ, but the most difficult to shut down. Imagery is the best way, so think of a beautiful place and walk across it, looking at everything as you go. Continue with the breathing and relaxing. Another visualisation is to count backwards from 40 – with each breath out for a number. If you lose your place, start again. The brain will soon get the message.

5. BE 'Quiet, Calm, and Peaceful': As you go about your day, watch how you behave. This is insight. People who

are anxious may talk a lot and raise their voices. This uses up a lot of energy, and if you are feeling exhausted, it will add to the problem. Try not to rush around. Walk slowly and deliberately, whilst checking your posture for round shoulders, etc. Leave other people to get on with their own lives, and try not to be at everyone's beck and call.

Eventually, with practise, you will be able to relax on demand, and any part of the five B's can be used whenever needed, for example, when driving, at work, shopping, or at home. Learning this method of relaxation will be a big help, as it can be used in any situation where anxiety levels rise.

Early waking from sleep was always said in psychiatry to be due to depression, but in homeopathy we describe it as more to do with 'anticipatory anxiety', which reflects worrying about what you have to do the next day.

Sleep research has revealed what happens to people when they are asleep, and has shown that dreams are part of normal sleep, and that night terrors are due to anxiety. Dreams and night terrors come out of your subconscious, and often reflect memories of things that are frightening.

The consequences of sleeping poorly are tiredness, exhaustion, and the brain not functioning at its proper level. During the day our anxieties are subjugated by our activities, but at night they can run free and express themselves in our dreams.

The solution to sleep problems is firstly to stop worrying about how much sleep you get. Focus on your days rather than your sleepless nights. Take five minutes during the day to be silent and disconnected. Practise breathing and relaxation techniques, things like yoga, and the five B's. Give yourself a digital curfew. Switch off televisions and mobile phones one hour before bed, and don't watch anxiety-provoking programmes. If you wake, do not get up to make tea, for example. Go to the toilet in the dark if possible, so that the light doesn't wake you up even more. Exercise during the day, but not in the evenings, except for yoga. Have a relaxing bath with Epsom salts that contain magnesium, which is a relaxant. Avoid alcohol near bedtime. Being awake is not the end of the world, so see it as an opportunity to breathe properly and meditate. Take-up hobbies like knitting, crocheting, or something calming and repetitive in the evening. Avoid watching television programmes with bad news, horror, crime, or fantasy. Watch more comedy and nature.

Emotional Eating

Stress causes an altered appetite. Eat your food mindfully. Don't eat and surf the Internet at the same time, for example. Eat slowly and chew well. Stop when you feel full. Keep track of your emotions and feelings before eating, to try to avoid snacking. Eat only at mealtimes. Resist the urge to gratify your feelings with food.

Music

Your taste in music can reflect your personality. Music comes in many genres, from classical to pop to country; there's music to dance to, to sing along with, but basically depends on rhythm, tempo, speed, and memorable tunes. There is a variety of music for everyone and a lot of people sing in choirs, which is very good for your mental health. There are more amateur orchestras in the UK than in most other countries. Learning to read music and play an orchestral instrument wires your brain up in a very healthy way. Dancing is also a good way of helping to improve your mental health.

Group drumming can reduce depression by nearly 40%, which is better than placebos or antidepressants (30% each). There is also a 20% reduction in anxiety levels. It improves social resilience and general mental well-being. Saliva samples taken from people during a trial of group drumming showed that their inflammatory processes in the immune system had also reduced.

This shows that getting out more, music, dancing, gardening, rambling, and going to concerts or the theatre are good for depression and anxiety. If you encourage these activities during childhood it makes a really good foundation for life. The more rock solid you make yourself mentally, the less life can knock you down. You are therefore more able to adapt to change. But we all need peace and quiet to let our brains calm down and settle. Taking part in a group activity increases your self-confidence. When you retire, join your local U3A (University of the third Age – the first 'age' being childhood and the second adulthood), which provides activities and friendship to keep you busy and active. Our local group has monthly talks, outings by coach, and many groups to join, from Latin and tap-dancing to gardening and rambling.

Music therapy has been used for people with mental health problems and learning disabilities in the Steiner schools since the 1920s. Nordoff and Robbins developed the techniques further more recently. As well as people with mental health problems and learning disabilities, it is also known to help people with dementia, as does art therapy.

Making Friends

Loneliness can be a real problem and not only for the elderly. The ability to mix with people depends on confidence, hearing, and self-esteem. It is much more common in women than men. Why do girls usually outperform boys at all levels of education, and yet go on to earn less, and occupy less senior posts? Their inner critic judges them to be not good enough. They can, therefore, lack self-confidence. It is very important to deal with this. You can tell yourself that no one cares if you wear the wrong shoes, and anyway, they are under the table so no one sees them. Social media can undermine this, so avoid it.

A lot of women feel as if they are frauds, permanently on the verge of being found out, which is called the imposter syndrome.

To silence your inner critic the trick is to accept that you can't be good at everything and that this doesn't matter. If you worry about it, it becomes an issue. We should teach young girls about failure, being bad at things, and that it is okay to not care about failure and go and be good at something else instead. J. K. Rowling said it is impossible to live without failing at something, unless you live so cautiously that you might as well not have lived at all, in which case you have failed by default. You should remember the comfort of ordinary things like walking, cooking, gardening, pets, cycling, etc. Ordinariness induces stability. Hobbies soothe the soul and give you a respite from the world. Laughter is the best medicine, so watch plenty of comedy!

There are many fears that anxious people suffer from not measuring up to others, being unable to cope, not having enough friends, being a failure compared to others, and from the emotions of envy and jealousy.

We shouldn't pressurise ourselves. We should take a more philosophical attitude – que sera sera!

Mindfulness and Meditation

Mindfulness is about paying attention to the present moment. If you think about where you are putting your keys down, for example, instead of rushing off to do the next thing, you will remember where you put them. Do not be hurried, too busy, or harassed, because this will make you forget. Do not rush your food or do something else at the same time as eating, and savour every mouthful.

If you are out on a walk, stop regularly to admire the scenery in silence. Do not talk so much. Do not try to do more than one thing at a time. Do not obsess about having the perfect body. No one has. Remember you have a limited supply of will power.

Feeling safe decreases anxiety levels. Wear nice colours to freshen up your soul, avoiding black, which can be depressing. Spending more time in nature improves self-esteem, as does looking at pictures of nature. Children should be taught to not care what people think of them in the way of teasing, bullying, and snide remarks because it reduces their self-confidence. They should do the opposite and feel sorry for the people whose behaviour is bad, as they are the ones with the problems.

Meditation is concentrating the mind on something you are thinking about, like going for a walk on a beach at sunset on a hot day, and watching the sun go down. You probably have a favourite beach, which makes the process easier. You silently watch other people and their dogs, say, and watch the waves and the sunset. If you become skilled at meditation you can actually empty your mind. Every time your mind wanders you gently bring it back to the beach. This makes the brain shut down and run at a more basic level, which is very restful and calming. If you meditate regularly, you can train your mind to be more present and to wander less, and you become less likely to be anxious and stressed. Ten minutes a day is enough.

Mental Health in Old Age

New and different worries happen as you get older. Surveys show that older people worry about loss of independence, declining health, running out of money, not being able to live at home any more, death of a spouse or other family member, inability to manage their own activities of daily living, not being able to drive any more, isolation or loneliness, being cared for by strangers, and fear of falling or hurting themselves.

Generally though, older people have lower levels of stress, as they've had a lifetime of experience in coping. They have different stresses to younger people, and do not get as exhausted from rushing around.

Cognitive Behavioural Therapy (CBT)

The brain is hardwired by life events, and thought patterns become embedded and difficult to alter or dislodge. There is no conventional medication to help under these circumstances. Cognitive behavioural therapy works to alter these patterns and replace them with more robust ways of thinking. Anger management is also a part of CBT. It can take a long time to achieve results with this therapy. Homeopathic treatment is much faster, and should be used in all departments of psychiatry.

You should try to identify what is causing your high stress levels and why you are not coping. Break it down into small parts and focus on one part at a time. Identify your fears and try the homeopathic remedy gelsemium, which has helped many people with anticipatory anxiety, like fear of flying.

Accept the past and try to move on. If you have post-traumatic stress disorder, see a homeopath who should be able to help.

Develop resilience, which means find good friends and see them outside school or work. Be interested in your schooling or job, and be happy.

If something is bothering you, try speaking about it to someone who will be supportive and make helpful suggestions.

Take-up yoga. 450 Dru yoga participants were asked about the effects of their practice. 72% said it reduced their back pain, 93% said it improved their spinal flexibility, 86% said it increased their energy levels, 89% noticed improved breathing, 89% could reduce and control their stress levels more easily, 81% developed greater confidence and self-empowerment, 84% had improved mood, 83% were emotionally more balanced, and 91% gained peace of mind by overcoming negative thinking. Perhaps it should be done in every school.

Anger

We all get angry at times, especially when things are not going the way we would like them to. It is not easy to take a step back and look at things differently. The trouble with anger, is that it causes chemical changes in the body and you can become ill as a result of this process. It raises the blood pressure and was always thought to cause strokes and heart attacks. Now, we are more interested in cholesterol levels.

Anger is related to anxiety in that it is the result of something disliked, and anxiety results in trying to change things. Doctors often cause a lot of anger and anxiety in patients, like with 'white coat syndrome', which can cause a rise in blood pressure. Anger often gets suppressed, as the system does not always seem to work in the patient's favour. The fact that people usually have to wait so long for test results makes them feel angry and/ or anxious. If a doctor does not have a good consultation with a patient, the patient might feel very angry. If things go wrong, the patient feels angry enough to make a complaint. Complaints departments are huge now, and need a lot of staff to service them, and take up a lot of time and money. This could be avoided if homeopathy was used more widely.

The medical students that I taught had to fill in a questionnaire at the end of the course. One of the subjects they frequently mentioned was case history taking, and how much it had improved with the homeopathy training. I understand that there is now a department in a local medical school to train doctors in empathy, which should relieve a lot of patients' anger. It is a pity that this sort of training is found necessary, and medical students are not chosen for their own empathetic abilities.

People should recognise anger in themselves and try to deal with it. They will not get any help from the medical profession. Anger management is usually for people with high levels of anger, but low or variable amounts are just as unhealthy over a long period of time.

To summarise, anxiety affects us all at sometime, but in individual ways. As the GP is either not going to recognise it in you, as they have been trained to only take into account your physical symptoms that relate to physical disease, and have no medication to help, or any time to give you advice, it is mainly up to you to realise what your problem is and try to deal with it yourself.

The most helpful thing you can do to feel more relaxed is mindfulness, which means reading your body for tension, and trying to stop your mind wandering by being in the present, or listening to music and maybe singing along. Walking in nature, especially near trees, is very calming... hug a tree! Reading is restful, but not newspapers, which can make you angry. Being alone and having a nice hot bath relaxes you, but make sure you only put natural perfumes in it. Being alone is restful if you have family members to look after. Try to find some time for yourself. Even daydreaming and watching TV is restful, as long as what you watch is calming.

If you feel stressed or restless try some of the suggestions above. It is probably the reason why so many people go around listening to music on their devices.

Life is so relentless and stressful that we should all be aware of the effect it is having on our bodies, and try to do something about it before it causes physical illness to stop you in your tracks.

14

THE VITAL FORCE

In Hahnemann's time there was no explanation of how the human body worked. In fact, scientists are just now beginning to put the parts together. The new disciplines of neuropsychiatry and psychoneurology are steps in the right direction. It is unlikely that there will be a psychocardiology department for sometime; even if, as a cardiologist, you see the progress that your neurology colleagues are making, there is usually very little co-operation between departments.

You would think that general practice would take the ideas on board, as it would give such insight into a person's illness, but GPs would need extra time to explore this idea in the 10-minute consultation time, although when I had been trained in homeopathy, I did it automatically, and it shortened the consultation time, as I was able to get to the crux of the consultation quickly.

It was the American physician, and forefather of modern homeopathy, James Tyler Kent who first wrote a book about symptoms, published in 1912. He realised that the brain was the most important organ in the body, and devoted the first, large chapter to it. Until I looked at this book, I had never realised the importance of the mind in the whole system. He gathered symptoms from doctors all over the world and the remedies that were known to have cured them. By doing this, he managed to increase our knowledge of the remedies considerably, and it has been only recently that this knowledge has been extended further by working out the basic properties of the groups, like minerals, plant and animal remedies.

I read about psycho-neuro-hormono-immunology and this put everything together and made sense of homeopathy as a whole-person discipline. It meant that someone's rheumatoid arthritis was not a disease of the joints but of a whole person. I also had to read up on nutrition, and learnt a lot when the Midlands' branch of the Faculty of Homeopathy invited Patrick Holford to give a day seminar. It is a pity that nutrition plays such a small part in the medical curriculum, as it plays such a large part in illness. There is no hope for a cure of an illness unless the doctor knows how illness is caused, and the patient is willing to change their habits. Now so much is known about diet and diabetes, you would think that all doctors would inform their patients that type 2 diabetes can be reversed if they stick to a low-carbohydrate diet. One patient with whom I discussed this said he was happy with the way things were (he was four stone overweight), and his blood sugars were fine as long as he took his tablets. He now has peripheral neuropathy and cannot walk.

It is very important to see people in a joined-up fashion. Who knows what influences, more or less, are governing patients' symptoms. It will of course be different for different people. This is why I find homeopathic practice so interesting. No matter how much inflammation there is in the body, and in which parts it is situated, homeopathy will help. The symptoms of an individual patient tell me all about them. The doctor has to interpret them to find the correct medicine. When that is found and taken there is a rapid alleviation of the whole illness. One Victorian homeopathic doctor said that there is a correct way to get better, and if the patient said they felt better in themself, and their joints were beginning to improve, then that was the correct direction of cure. There is no similar pattern looked for in conventional medicine, as the doctor is only interested in the joints.

It was Samuel Hahnemann who first used the expression 'vital force'. He knew nothing of the information we now have about patients, gleaned from blood tests and scans. In his book *Organon of Medicine*, an 'organon' being an instrument or tool, he said that the vital force is the unseen, subconscious, automatic, self-regulating, and self-sustaining invisible part of the body. Now we can measure hormone levels and inflammatory markers and see which parts of the brain are damaged. This does not tell you how well the patient's system is actually working.

This is your vital force. It reflects how all your systems cope with the constant changes that take place – for example, the number of cells that turn cancerous every day, the number of organisms that infect you regularly, and how well you cope with stressful events.

Hahnemann worked out that the health of your vital systems was dependent on your nutrition. He said that when a person falls ill the vital force becomes untuned by the dynamic influence of the hostile disease agent. It is quite something to talk about the body in these terms in 1810, when the book was first published. He wondered how the vital force makes the body produce symptoms, and although we now know about genes and various chemicals in the body, this fundamental question still eludes us.

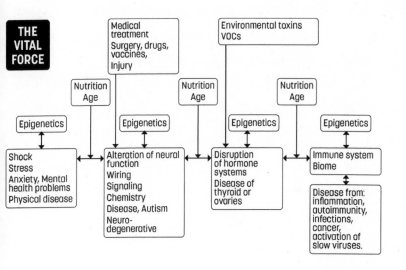

He also said that treating symptoms with opposites, that is, chemicals which suppress symptoms, only makes them return when the medicine is stopped or the body becomes accustomed to the chemical. Disease must be treated with similar, that is, a medicine made from a substance whose poisoning symptoms are most similar to the patient's symptoms.

The chart above is a visual explanation of how the body works. It shows the relationship between all the functions of the body. If everything is connected to everything, looking at individual pieces of information is not so useful. The system is a feedback, so that all connections know what is in or out of balance, and can make the appropriate adjustments. It also shows that one part is not more important than any other, and never functions in isolation.

It is important to ask the patient how they feel. You will soon get the information you need. Whether they feel better, about the same, or worse, is most of what you need to know. It is rare to be asked this question now.

It would seem from the chart, which is a summary of what has been written so far, that all disease has its origin in the mind. In other words, your actions and thoughts are what cause disease. This starts with the foetus and continues all the way through life. Everything you think or do has an effect on the body. It may be minor and easily healed, but if it is deep-rooted, severe, or repeated, it will have a lasting effect. Your vital force is damaged and untuned. The consequences may be a cold or minor illness, but if your 'VF' is badly damaged then a physical illness like rheumatoid arthritis may show itself. This will depend on which genes are switched. Genes are never a cause of illness; they just determine which illness you get.

This is why we need to look after as many parts of the system as we can, mainly by paying attention to diet and anxieties. If we understand how the system is working and how it fails, we will be good at fundamentally preventing illness.

15

CONCLUSIONS

All this may seem very gloomy, as if everything is stacked against you if you have to deal with an illness. Most of the time there are no problems, but I hear too many stories of things that go wrong to be complacent. It seems as if the present situation is evolving back to a time of self-reliance for health. Consequently, many people try to look after themselves when it comes to looking for answers, often using the Internet. Are there any alternatives?

If you have an emergency, the paramedics are wonderful. It is what happens afterwards that may cause problems. Some of the emergency services are outsourced to private companies to try to save money. The NHS is stretched to its limit and running out of money and staff. You would think that under these circumstances they would be glad of any help that they were offered. Why are they so hostile to other forms of therapy, like hypnosis, acupuncture, osteopathy, and homeopathy? Hypnosis and osteopathy are not a threat, as they do not involve medication, and doctors can use these practices in their surgeries if the patient is willing, and if there is time!

Homeopathy can be seen as a threat, however, because it involves medication and the patients do well. Once a doctor uses it in GP, word gets around and patients request it. If this idea spread, where would it end? The answer is that the drug companies' sales would be much reduced.

If most of the NHS were homeopathic, as is the case in the public healthcare system in parts of India, doctors and nurses would need considerable retraining. In India, the situation for medical students is that they either go to medical school to learn the homeopathic method or conventional prescribing. There are plenty of medical schools that teach only the homeopathic method. That does not mean that patients who choose a homeopathic hospital miss out on investigations, like endoscopies and scans, or treatment with surgery. It would only mean that the medication would be homeopathic.

In fact, it would be possible to introduce small numbers of medicines to each department in the NHS, like aconite for shock, arnica for injury, and symphytum for bone-healing, into A & E. The complex theory and practice of homeopathy is not needed at this level. There would never be any problem with these remedies interfering with any medication that the patient was already taking, nor any harm to the patient from the remedies if they needed surgery.

Arnica could also be available in post-operative wards. I asked my ladies who were going in for a hysterectomy to take some arnica with them to use when they came round from the anaesthetic. The next day the nurse would do a round, asking what pain relief people wanted. My ladies always said none, because of the arnica. The nurse always knew who the doctor responsible for this outcome was, but no one ever asked me to go to talk to them about it.

However, one day I had to go to the GP labour ward to see a lady who needed a complicated repair. I said I would give her some of the arnica I always carried around with me in my bag. The nurse said that there was already some in the cupboard that other GPs used, and would give her some. GP labour wards no longer exist.

The knock-on effect would be that lots of money would be saved, as patients would be out of pain very rapidly and would heal quickly. All post-operative and post-partum patients should have arnica, and this would reduce the amount of analgesics prescribed. The only losers, again, would be big pharma.

We all know that antibiotics do not always treat infections, because some bacteria have become resistant to them. If all patients who have urinary infections, for example, were treated with D-mannose and homeopathic remedies instead, there would rarely be any need for antibiotics. Other problems like acne, tonsillitis and ear infections are also easily treated with homeopathy. In fact, the infections stop happening when homeopathic remedies are used.

The treatment of pneumonia with homeopathy before the arrival of antibiotics produced considerably better results than conventional medicine. 50% died in London's hospitals, but only 2% died in the homeopathic hospital, with similar outcomes when treating cholera. Remedies are made from all the bacteria, like MRSA, and can be given in conjunction with other medical treatment. Should all doctors not have a duty to their patients to find out what will help them?

The problem is much more difficult when chronic disease is the diagnosis. There are now hundreds of homeopathic remedies, and to choose the correct one needs a lot of studying. Does the patient need a plant, animal, or mineral remedy, and in which potency? There has been a lot written about this recently, particularly by Indian doctors. Homeopathy is not stuck in Victorian times, and remedies and prescribing patterns have changed and have been updated.

To cure a patient of a chronic disease means trying to find out what is at the basis of the illness in this particular patient. The search is for the constitutional remedy: the one that matches the person's individual responses. Conventional medicine just treats the symptoms, or attempts to suppress the immune-system response occurring.

Mineral remedies are taken from every element in the periodic table, plus all their compounds. Compounds like natrum muriaticum (common salt), have been used for many years. A substance like salt is not poisonous in small amounts, but in large amounts it is. Natrum mur. is a frequently used remedy for the effects of grief. Psychologists, psychiatrists and GPs could find this remedy very helpful. Sulphur is a possible remedy for eczema. However, it is necessary to learn the principles of prescribing minerals, which depend on the row and column in which the element is found in the periodic table, and whether or not a compound is needed, or just the element. Arsenicum album is a commonly used medicine for anticipatory anxiety, whereas natrum mur. is used for suppressed anger, along with many other remedies.

Plant remedies are numerous. For example, we have already heard of belladonna, which was given to a child with tonsillitis, and also to one with Tourette's syndrome. These two did have one thing in common – streptococcus.

There are 33 families of plants used in homeopathy, some having nine plants in use in each. It is very possible that there are more plants waiting to be discovered for their benefits with regard to homeopathy. Some plants are used more in certain countries, which reflects the environment in which they grow, which also reflects where the patients live and may alter their disease patterns.

Animal remedies are a big group, including spiders, snakes, mammals, insects, birds, and molluscs. All have poisoning effects that reflect characteristics, which also reflect patients' behaviour and mannerisms.

There are levels of case-history taking, starting at the surface, which is the patient's name, details and symptoms. Next are emotions, then delusions, and finally sensations, which are symptoms from the deepest level that the patient experiences. It is rare to get to the deepest level, and needs a lot of experience to get someone to tell you about it.

A man of 60 had Forestier's disease of the spine and ligaments. He'd already had both knees and hips replaced and his spine was fusing. He had good and bad days, when his mobility was poor or a bit better. He used to do martial arts and now felt powerless, and wanted to give up the fight. He also had mild diabetes. The conventional treatment of non-steroidal anti-inflammatory drugs had been no help. He talked a lot about immobility – what it meant to him, and how it affected him. His hobby had been long-distance walking.

During the homeopathic consultation he was in a situation where he was talking about things that no one had asked him before. It turned out that he was petrified by immobility and it panicked him. He imagined himself confined to a wheelchair, then a bed, and not being able to do the basic things needed in order to survive. He blamed all his symptoms on himself, and therefore needed a mineral remedy. The remedy chosen was niccolum, and given as 30C daily until his follow-up appointment two months later.

At his next appointment he had lost weight and his diabetes was much more controlled. His pain and stiffness were considerably better, and he was sleeping for eight hours rather than his usual four. Subsequently, he was much better in himself and there was no further deterioration in his spine.

This private consultation took two hours. The patient got a very helpful outcome. If he had seen a specialist in rheumatology, there would have been a diagnosis but no guarantee of any improvement. Homeopathic specialists have to do the same amount of rigorous postgraduate training as a conventional specialist in order to get their MFHom degree. It usually takes three years or longer. To become a fellow, you are elected by the Fellows Committee, having proved your worth to them and the Faculty, in my case by the study of haemophilia patients.

It can be very difficult to find the right remedy, but it can also be very easy. A lady in her 60s came to see me because of an attack of bronchitis that would not clear up. The whole thing was too much for her, and she was tearful and felt helpless. She'd had a number of similar attacks after colds, and a deep, loose cough, which troubled her at night and first thing in the morning. She also had catarrh and thick, yellowy-green sputum. She could not bear to be in a hot, stuffy room. Every time she coughed she passed some urine.

It did not take long (we only had 5-minute appointments, and had to fit extras in as well) to decide to give her pulsatilla, the wind flower, which cleared her cough in two days, after spending both days coughing much more sputum up than usual. Antibiotics were not needed.

Psychiatry

At a conference in Dubai, a psychiatrist, Dr Zafeiriou, stated that homeopathy can reduce the duration of hospitalisation, quantity of medication needed, number of laboratory examinations, frequency of relapses, and the individual and state healthcare costs. He also said it improves overall health, helps all chronic diseases, excluding irreversible tissue damage, has no side effects, and can be successfully combined with any other kind of treatment. It can also help behavioural problems, including those of prisoners and offenders, as well as children. He called upon the mental healthcare community to adopt homeopathy as a tool to treat psychiatric disorders, and to move away from conventional medicines that can sometimes have severe side effects.

Dr Zafeiriou said that in psychiatry there are no medicines designed to be curative – just those that relieve symptoms. Homeopathy can treat all kinds of disorders, from anxiety and phobias, to depression and schizophrenia. In mental hospitals, homeopathy can treat patients with severe mental disorders, contributing considerably to the therapeutic outcome of conventional psychiatric treatment.

Modern medicine has a plethora of techniques to use for diagnoses – so many, in fact, that doctors barely lay hands on patients, especially in obstetrics. Scanning techniques were invented after World War II by a doctor who had worked with radar imaging. He was keen to try it out on women who had bled during pregnancy, to locate the position of the placenta. In the last 50 years, it has developed into an investigation which has been used so routinely that nobody thinks of the consequences.

If a patient is having radiotherapy, homeopaths advise them to take radium bromide 30C, a medicine made from water and alcohol exposed to radium, which is then succussed. It always seemed to help prevent skin damage in breast cancer treated with radiotherapy. Perhaps people should try ultrasound 30C to counteract ultrasound damage, and X-ray 30C if frequent X-rays are needed. This advice should be suggested to people who work in scanning, radiotherapy, and X-ray departments.

If people are unhappy with – or damaged by – modern medicine, there is no reason why they should not take advice from other disciplines. The only problem is cost. Insurance companies prefer standard advice, which is very costly. Perhaps they could be persuaded to look at the alternatives. In my private practice, patients were usually covered by their medical insurance – until more recently.

The Chief Medical Officer has said that everyone should look at alternative treatments to take the strain off the NHS, and if insurance companies would start paying for consultations and treatment again, it would cost a lot less and be effective. The losers would be the consultants who do private practice and get paid a lot for it. There would, however, be happier, healthier patients, and that is what being a doctor is all about.

Scottish doctors train in homeopathy at the NHS Centre for Integrative Care, formerly the Glasgow Homeopathic Hospital, and have not been stopped from prescribing remedies as English ones have. Their individual prescribing costs will be lower than in England, as mine were in our practice. This would release money that could be used elsewhere, for example in social services, if carried out in England.

It is time for a change in thinking, and to see homeopathy as a system that has a lot of advantages which could be integrated into the NHS.

If all patients, particularly those with small children, kept a homeopathic first aid kit at home, then they would rarely need to consult a doctor. My mentor, Dr R. A. F. Jack, used to prescribe a few remedies for each new mum to keep in the house. He rarely had to go out on visits to see the children. This could be translated into A & E attendances. It would do no harm to give each child with a temperature aconite, whilst waiting to see a doctor. If the parents had aconite at home, it would save a trip to A & E.

It would be a lot cheaper to provide aconite on prescription than it would to be seen in hospital.

Dr Jack would give each new patient, on registration, written advice on an instructions sheet. When all prescriptions were free of charge, some remedies from the list were prescribed. As charges are now, it would be cheaper to buy them yourself from the manufacturers.

All first aid kits should contain arnica and aconite.

David's Story:
As Told By David's Mum

David has a dual diagnosis of Down's syndrome and autism. In addition, he has severe learning disabilities and challenging behaviour. He is an extremely complex young man who can easily be misunderstood, and over- or under-judged for his ability, understanding, and health.

He struggles to identify where he is injured or feeling ill. He will always say he has a headache, sore throat, or tummy ache, regardless of where he is hurting. Carers need to use a process of elimination to discover the real cause of his pain. Because David does not react or respond to pain in the way we do, it is easy to assume he is okay or not in pain. Medical professionals often have the same problem and have missed injuries in the past. The more time you spend with David, the more you really get to know and understand him, rather than just support his physical needs, and the easier it gets to pick up on what is really wrong with him.

David has had six surgeries: open-heart surgery, one undescended testicle, two hernia repairs, an appendectomy, and a tonsillectomy.

He has been assessed by a psychologist and was found to display depressive tendencies, and sometimes he refuses to participate in activities that he would usually enjoy. David undertook an initial Mini PAS-ADD Interview (Psychiatric Assessment Schedule for Adults with Developmental Disabilities). The outcome of the initial test indicated that David had a tendency towards depressive disorder, which is still the case to date. It is therefore very important that 'chat times' are always available and fully utilised to help David address things that are causing him worry and anxiety, before he slides into a depressive mood. Chat time is a one-to-one session with a staff member of David's choice in a quiet environment.

In common with a lot of people with DS, David has had heart surgery, which has left him with a leaking valve. He also has a knee which easily dislocates, and there is already extensive damage to it. He also has sleep apnoea and uses a CPAP breathing machine at night.

For several years, David had prolonged periods of yellow, loose stools. The GP always said it was IBS, probably from anxiety and stress. His mum monitored all bowel activity and compared it with his food intake.

It seemed obvious that the problem was gluten, as any gluten in his diet saw a dramatic change in the colour and consistency of his stools and upper gastric pain. If we totally eliminated gluten from his diet, after 72 hours his stools became brown and firm again. However, any cross-contamination, as simple as holding hands with someone who had eaten a sandwich, seemed to bring on loose stools again. David was referred to an immunologist after three months of having two loperamide every morning, and then as required, meaning he averaged 109 loperamide tablets a month, but still averaged over 180 bowel movements a month. A coeliac blood test always came back negative. The doctor therefore did not think that David's bowel problem was due to gluten intolerance.

Also, his thyroid-stimulating hormone level was low, and his T3 and T4 levels were off the charts, so the doctor said that he needed urgent assessment and referral for thyroid treatment. (This was annoying, as she had been asking for further investigations on and off for eight years, and was always only given TSH tests, which came back at the low end of normal, so no further investigations were done.) David's T3 and T4 levels show a huge thyroid problem, which causes fatigue, lack of attention, and diarrhoea.

Because his vitamin D levels are so low, he has a problem with tiredness and fatigue, cardiac and pulmonary function, brain activity, his endocrine system, and a massive problem with his digestive system. His body finds it very hard to absorb nutrients, and his brain overloads with sugar, which it then dumps into his body and turns to fat, so with low vitamin D levels you can't lose weight easily, and could see weight gain even on a restricted or modified diet.

Because David isn't getting the right nutrients, his body is keeping some food in his system for too long (that would explain why after 12 hours of no food or drink, when he had an endoscopy there was food sitting in his tummy); this produces gases and toxins that poison the body, causing diarrhoea. Also, some foods the body deems as waste will be forced through the digestive system at a fast rate, causing more diarrhoea. Gluten is one of the hardest substances for the body to process, and as David's body keeps it for too long, he reacts as if he were gluten-intolerant.

The sweeteners in diet drinks and in fat-free yoghurts (Slimming World staples) can cause diarrhoea if you have low vitamin D levels.

David's thyroid issues turned out to be acute thyroiditis, but now he has normal read-outs again. His next problem, however, was headaches.

He would sit and hold his head, and moan or yell with pain. Sitting quietly did not alleviate it, nor did paracetamol. It escalated to the point where he had to go to A & E, but the doctors could not diagnose the problem, so he was sent home with strong painkillers.

At this point his medication list was esomeprazole, vitamin D, lisinopril, paracetamol, ibuprofen, loperamide, co-codamol, diazepam, and sumatriptan for his severe headaches.

The next terrible occurrence for David was a seizure, so he ended up in A & E again. He was put under the care of the epilepsy nurse, who told his mum that everyone was entitled to one unexplained seizure!

Some months later he had another fit, and was seen at a different A & E. He was given analgesia, and, as he seemed to be a bit better, was sent home with an appointment for two weeks hence. Before then there was another trip to the GP who said to continue with his medication. However, he had a long, major seizure a few days later, so went in an ambulance to A & E, as the fit had not subsided. They decided that it was caused by another migraine and wanted to send him home. His mum called for the learning disability nurse, who came to assess David's situation. She asked for him to be seen by a neurologist, who admitted David to a ward and put him on an analgesic drip. David's blood tests and brain scan were normal so he was discharged; but he kept saying, 'too much pain!' whilst holding his head. While in the ward, David had further fits, which his mum recorded on her phone. She felt the staff did not really believe her story about what was going on. A portable EEG (electro-encephalogram) was done. As the equipment had to be moved from another hospital it took hours, and David had settled a bit.

The next day he was seen by a doctor who had experience of treating epilepsy in people with Down's syndrome. He checked David's results and said that the X-ray showed signs of considerable damage to his sinuses, which are very underdeveloped in people with DS. So it transpired that a severe and long-lasting sinus infection had given David so much pain that he eventually had fits as a result. Obviously antibiotics were prescribed to solve the problem, so David went home with a two-week course of the antibiotic clarithromycin. However, he was only a bit better after the course...

David's mum told me all that had happened to him when I was acting as MO for the Side by Side Theatre Company, a local charity for adults with learning disabilities, who put on a show annually. David was taking part, albeit very lethargically. His mum came to sit with me during one of the practices, and explained all of his past history, and what the situation was at that time. I asked her to bring him to see me the following day, which she did, and I gave him three tablets of the homeopathic remedy medorrhinum.

The response was amazing. He discharged pus and blood from his nose for two days. It would seem that if he'd not had my treatment, the antibiotics would have only been a temporary relief. After another few days he told his mum he was better. He also stopped needing his night-time equipment for sleep apnoea, and had no more fits. I suggested that David's biome was damaged (probably by the esomeprazole), and that he should take some live-bacteria capsules.

You can make up your own mind about what this case reflects. All hospitals should have a learning disability nurse to look out for the rights of people with LD. Why do doctors not believe patients? Why are doctors not knowledgeable about Down's syndrome? Why does each hospital not have a specialist in homeopathy?

Knowing about the basics of medicine saves lives and money, as doctors make better diagnoses and ask for fewer investigations. In David's case it would have saved him months of ill health, pain, and unhappiness.

Doctors seem too tired or stressed out to try to learn new things, but the best investment I made was to go on the introductory course in homeopathy, and follow it up with more study and the MFHom examination. Courses are available via the Faculty of Homeopathy at the Royal London Hospital for Integrated Medicine in Great Ormond Street.

Patients need to ask their GPs to recommend a homeopath in the area that has good training and reliable results, via outcome studies. Look on the Faculty of Homeopathy website for MFHom-qualified doctors. There seems to be no possibility of the NHS embracing homeopathy as long as the manufacturers of drugs have their way, because a lot of research is funded by drug companies. Therefore, patients are often left to their own devices to find solutions to their problems. You will never regret using homeopathy.

Instructions for Taking Homeopathic Medicines

1. Homeopathic medicines are pleasant-tasting and should be sucked or chewed.

2. They can be given to people of any age or weight, during pregnancy, or to animals; and the dose is the same for all cases. Tablets can be crushed between spoons or dissolved in water, and then sipped or given from a spoon. If frequent doses are needed then dissolve two tablets in water, and take a dose as required.

3. Homeopathic medicines do not deteriorate and will keep their strength for years, despite their use-by date.

4. They can never be poisonous. A child could swallow a whole bottle of them and come to no harm. The medication will only work if the person is ill and actually needs the remedy in the bottle, in which case it heals.

5. The medicines have never been tested on animals – only humans of all ages.

6. Homeopathic medicines can be taken with prescribed or over-the-counter medicines, and do not interfere with their actions. They should be taken before food or drink.

7. In the rare case of an aggravation of symptoms occurring, that is, the symptoms getting worse, stop the medication and wait. It is usually a sign that the remedy is correct and working well. Symptoms usually subside rapidly and improvement sets in.

8. If you buy your own homeopathic medicines, ask for the 30C strength. Take the dosage for the remedies below as described. You cannot take too much of them, however, because when you feel better you forget to take them and that is correct. If any symptoms come back though, or do not seem better, then another tablet can be sucked. Once you *are* better, you will stay well without having to take more. Some suggestions are below.

Aconite: For shock, anxiety, croup, or a fever. After a shock, which causes fear; also for panic attacks, palpitations, trembling, feeling restless, anxious, or afraid. At the onset of a fever; the patient feels cold, but their skin is very warm to the touch. Also for the onset of croup.

Dosage: Suck one dose every five minutes until relief, then as required.

Arnica: For injuries, including sprains, fractures (also take symphytum to heal bones), kicks, blows, bruises, concussion, and general accidents. Also for muscular tiredness after journeys and sports, and after surgery, dental work, and childbirth.

Dosage: Suck one dose every hour until relief, then as required.

Arsenicum Album: Do not be concerned by the name of this medication. It is indeed white arsenic, but can never do any harm because of the way that this remedy is made. If you gave the tablets to a public health analyst they would not actually find any arsenic in them. They could not measure the energy in the remedy.

Dosage: One 3x a day for two days; one 2x a day for two days; then one daily.

The main problems that arsenicum album is used for are sickness and diarrhoea at the same time, causing severe weakness. I once cured a man with this remedy in 30 minutes. He had been stranded in the bathroom with a bowl on his knees. He took the arsenicum and was well enough to go to an important meeting the same afternoon.

It is also one of the remedies for anticipatory anxiety, when a person is restless from anxiety, and sometimes has a fear of death and of being left alone. People who need this remedy are fastidious and insecure. They feel very cold, exhausted and have burning pains. They sit and fidget, and can never relax because they are always worrying.

Belladonna: For high fevers when a person is red and flushed, feels burning hot, and may be delirious. Effective for children with a history of febrile convulsions as well. Helpful if someone has an inability to swallow with a sore throat. Also for a throbbing pain, such as migraines, headaches, and boils.

Dosage: One dose every 15 minutes until relief.

Bryonia: For painful joints, and where pain gets worse with any movement, including headaches and painful coughs. The person feels irritable and wants to be left alone in the quiet. They can be thirsty for cold drinks and the affected part often feels better if pressure is applied or if it's lain on.

Dosage: One dose every 15 minutes until relief.

Cantharis: For cystitis and burns. For an attack of cystitis with burning pain take with D-mannose every time you need the toilet. You should be able to avoid antibiotics.

Dosage: For burns, apply cold water and take cantharis every ten minutes until the burn is less painful, then keep reducing the dose and take until better.

Carbo Veg: For wind, either in the abdomen or released. The stomach feels distended and clothing needs to be loosened.

Dosage: One dose as needed.

Chamomilla: For frantic pain such as teething, where one cheek can be red, and there may be diarrhoea; the child is angry and impatient. Also for any unbearable pain like earache.

Dosage: One dose every five minutes until relief.

Colocynth: For abdominal colic in babies or adults with IBS. The pain is usually better when doubling up and applying heat. It gets worse when getting worked up or angry.

Dosage: One dose every 15 minutes as required.

Drosera: For coughing followed by vomiting. Spasms of coughing. A dry, irritating cough that gets worse when lying down, getting warm in bed, drinking, laughing, and at night.

Dosage: One dose every 10 minutes as required.

Ferrum Phos: For mild fevers, and the onset of flu, colds, earache, or a sore throat.

Dosage: One dose every 15 minutes until relief.

Gelsemium: For nerves, tension-related pain, and flu. Also good for anticipatory anxiety for things like stage fright, driving tests, exams, flying, etc. Helps tension headaches and neck pain, and the onset of flu with lethargy, headache, fever, aching muscles, and sore throat.

Dosage: One dose every 30 minutes until relief.

Ignatia: For grief, and the early stages of a loss or bereavement, when very tearful and emotional.

Dosage: Suck one when required.

Ipecac: For wheezy coughs, when the chest feels tight, especially if nausea is present. Also helps nose bleeds.

Dosage: One dose as often as required.

Ledum: For puncture wounds, including injections, insect stings, pin pricks, needles, etc. Ledum prevents infection and allergies.

Dosage: Take a dose as soon as you can, and repeat as necessary.

Nat Mur: For cold sores, and the onset of colds with sneezing and a runny nose. This remedy is also used for depression, acne, and migraines, but you need to consult a practitioner, because there are also many other remedies for these problems.

Dosage: One dose every 2 hours for the first six doses, then one dose as required.

Phosphorus: For vomiting and laryngitis; the latter causing a hoarse voice, pain when talking, a tight chest, tickling cough, and craving for cold drinks.

Dosage: One dose as often as required for laryngitis. For repeated vomiting, as with gastric flu, take one dose after vomiting.

Pulsatilla: For catarrh, with sticky eyes, thick, coloured nasal catarrh, and a loose, rattly cough. Also for a blocked nose, loss of smell, and a lack of thirst, which usually improve in the open air, and get worse in a stuffy room.

Dosage: One dose every two hours until relief.

Rhus Tox: For shingles, cold sores, and rheumatism. The latter causes painful, stiff muscles and joints that get worse when sitting still, after which, the first movements are painful, but improve with limbering up; they also get worse in cold or wet weather. Take this remedy after arnica for a sprain with stiff muscles, as well as for flu with stiff muscles.

Dosage: One dose every 2 hours for the first six doses, then one dose as required.

Spongia: For a barking cough that is hard and painful, and sounds like a sea lion, usually due to croup, which is a viral infection. If your child has repeated attacks of croup, keep aconite and spongia in the house.

Dosage: As soon as the cough starts, usually in the night, give a dose of aconite followed by spongia. Repeat these doses every five minutes at first, then as the attack begins to improve, reduce their frequency. After using this regime, the attacks of croup will stop happening.

Many years ago, a paediatrician in a Welsh hospital treated all his admissions for croup with these medications. He gave the family a small bottle of each to take home. There were only ever two readmissions for croup, and they'd forgotten that they had some medication at home, so had not used it.

If you want to know whether your problem can be treated with a homeopathic method, then the answer is YES. There is plenty of information online, including individual case histories. If the situation is complicated, it is best to consult an experienced practitioner. It is, however, easy to obtain a small collection of remedies that will help with first aid.

The Queen is said to have taken her collection of remedies with her wherever she went. If a problem arose, her homeopathic physician was consulted by phone, and a remedy suggested.

Homeopathic medicines can be bought online very cheaply and easily, and once in your first aid kit, they'll never need to be replaced unless you run out, which is rare. Your family will be much healthier for it!

Online homeopathic pharmacies include:

Ainsworths (London); Freeman's (Glasgow); Helios (Tunbridge Wells); HomeoForce (Guernsey); Nelsons (London); Weleda (Ilkeston).